A Publication of the National Institute for the Psychotherapies

PSYCHOLOGICAL ASPECTS OF PREGNANCY, BIRTHING, AND BONDING

EDITED BY

BARBARA L. BLUM, Ph.D.

with
James L. Fosshage, Ph.D.
Kenneth A. Frank, Ph.D.
Henry Grayson, Ph.D.
Clemens A. Loew, Ph.D.
Henry Lowenheim, Ph.D.

VOLUME IV IN THE SERIES
NEW DIRECTIONS IN PSYCHOTHERAPY
Series Editor
PAUL OLSEN, Ph.D.

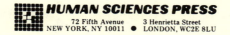 **HUMAN SCIENCES PRESS**
72 Fifth Avenue   3 Henrietta Street
NEW YORK, NY 10011 ● LONDON, WC2E 8LU

Copyright © 1980 by Human Sciences Press Inc. 72 Fifth Avenue,
New York, New York 10011

Printed in the United States of America

0123456789 987654321

Library of Congress Cataloging in Publication Data
Main entry under title:

Psychological aspects of pregnancy, birthing, and bonding.

(New directions in psychotherapy; v. 4)
At head of title: A publication of the National Institute for the Psychotherapies.
"Developed from a conference entitled 'the birth of an American child' that was
held in New York City on May 6, 1978."
Bibliography
Includes index.
1. Pregnancy—Psychological aspects—Congresses.
2. Childbirth—Psychological aspects—Congresses.
3. Mother and Child—Congresses. I. Blum, Barbara L.
II. National Institute for the Psychotherapies.
III. Series. [DNLM: 1. Pregnancy—Congresses.
2. Labor—Congresses. 3. Psychology—Congresses.
4. Parent–child relations—Congresses. W1 NE374FE
v. 4 / WQ200 P974 1978]
RG560.P79   155.6'46   LC 80–14227
ISBN 0–87705–210–7

CONTENTS

128926

To my mother
Ruth Blum Adler,
and to the memory of my father
Philip Leonard Blum

PREFACE

This book developed from a conference entitled *The Birth of an American Child* that was held in New York City on May 6, 1978. The purpose of this conference, which was sponsored by the National Institute for the Psychotherapies, was to study psychological and sociocultural factors which affect responses of prospective parents, their families, professionals, and society at large to pregnancy and childbirth. The participants represented professions including psychology, social work, medicine (obstetrics and gynecology, pediatrics, psychiatry), nursing, and education. The result was a unique interdisciplinary dialogue. The excellent response to this conference, the requests for copies of talks, and the absence of an interdisciplinary book on the psychological variables affecting pregnancy and childbirth experiences were major factors affecting the decision of the National Institute for the Psychotherapies to sponsor this volume. Most of the papers in this book are based on talks or workshops that were specifically prepared for the conference;

others are new and have not been previously presented or published. All represent the work of distinguished members of their respective professions.

B. L. B. 5/79

ACKNOWLEDGMENTS

I want to extend special gratitude to Dr. Alan R. Fleischman who, as program co-coordinator, helped develop *The Birth of an American Child* conference and solicit the participation of prominent members of the medical profession. His professional competence and dedication and his personal warmth were inspirations.

Thanks also are given to the Board of Directors of the National Institute for the Psychotherapies (N.I.P.), with special appreciation to Dr. Paul Olsen, Director of Publications, who, as liason with Human Sciences Press and with the N.I.P. office staff, gave freely of his time and expertise; to Dr. Henry Grayson, Executive Director, for his contagious enthusiasm, his faith, and his valued friendship; and to Dr. James Fosshage, Director of Clinical Research, for his sincere caring.

Gratitude also is due to the office staff of N.I.P. especially Ms. Karen Wachsman, Mr. Ralph Di Libero, Mr. Peter Funkhouser, and Ms. Sara Fleischer for their patient help in organizing the correspondence and paperwork involved in the preparation of this manuscript, and to Ms. Elsie Romero of Lehman College, City University of New York, for xeroxing and retyping many pages many times.

Finally, loving thanks to my dear, supporting, and encouraging friends, persons who have experienced some of my own rebirths, especially Drs. Jerome Kosseff, Elizabeth Thorne, and Tina Harrell; Ms. Linda Fleischman, and Ms. Ellen Epstein.

CONTRIBUTORS

BARBARA L. BLUM, PH.D., EDITOR, is Coordinator of Conferences at the National Institute for the Psychotherapies and on the faculty of the Department of Psychology at Herbert H. Lehman College, City University of New York. She is in private practice in New York City where she conducts comprehensive psychotherapy with adolescents and adults.

STEPHEN PAUL ADLER, PH.D., a practicing psychoanalyst, is on the faculty of, and intern coordinator at the National Psychological Association for Psychoanalysis. He also is on the faculty of the Center for Expressive Analysis, and is a Consultant to The Wholistic Childbirth Preparation and Family Center of New York.

MAXINE ANTELL-BUCKLEY, PH.D., is an Assistant Clinical Professor of Psychiatry and Supervising Psychologist at the Albert Einstein College of Medicine in New York. She also is in private practice.

LAURA BARBANEL, ED.D., is the Program Head of the Graduate Program in School Psychology at Brooklyn College, City University of New York. She was a member of the American Psychological Association Task Force on Sexism in Graduate Education in Psychology and is currently secretary of the Division of Psychotherapy of the American Psychological Association. She is in private practice in Brooklyn, New York.

HARRIET R. BARRY is a certified childbirth educator and a certified teacher of the Alexander Technique. She is in private practice and on the staff of Brookdale Medical Center, New York, and the faculty of The Life Institute, New York. She is co-founder of the Wholistic Childbirth Preparation and Family Center of New York.

ALICE EICHHOLZ, PH.D., is an Assistant Professor in the Department of Special Programs at Queens College, City University of New York, and a Research Associate at the Institute of Psychohistory. As a professional consultant in human relations and genealogy, she has published several books, the most recent of which is coauthored with James M. Rose entitled *Black Genesis* (Gale Research, 1978).

PHIMA ENGELSTEIN, PH.D., is Assistant Professor of Psychiatry in psychology at Albert Einstein College of Medicine and Head Psychologist at the Adult Outpatient Psychiatric Clinic at Jacobi Hospital in New York. She also is a member of the family therapy faculty with special interests in the future of the family and effects of pregnancy on the marital relationship. Her current research is on the psychological concomitants of artificial insemination. She has a private practice in individual and family therapy.

ALAN R. FLEISCHMAN, M.D., is Director, Division of Neonatology, Montefiore Hospital and Medical Center and The North Central Bronx Hospital, and is an Associate Professor of

Pediatrics at The Albert Einstein College of Medicine, Bronx, New York. He has published extensively in the areas of perinatal physiology, infant nutrition, and mineral metabolsim in infants and children.

DONNA SANDS FRYD, M.A. C.S.W., is a Medical Social Worker, Division of Neonatology, Department of Social Services, The North Central Bronx Hospital, New York.

DORIS HAIRE is President of the American Foundation of Maternal and Child Health, Inc. and Chair of the Committee of Health, Law and Regulation of both the International Childbirth Education Association and the National Woman's Health Network. Among her books and articles are *Implimenting Family Centered Maternal Care, The Cultural Warping of Childbirth* and *The Pregnant Patient's Bill of Rights*. She also is a well-known fetal advocate.

DAVID KLIOT, M.D., is Chairman of the New York City chapter of the American Society for Psychoprophylaxis in Obstetrics, Physicians' Division; Assistant Clinical Professor in the Department of Obstetrics and Gynecology at the State University of New York Downstate Medical Center; and Coordinator of the Childbirth Education Program at Brookdale Hospital Medical Center. He also serves as Obstetrical Consultant for the New York City Department of Health. He is currently investigating and quantifying the effects of childbirth techniques on parent–infant bonding.

HAZELANNE LEWIS, B. SOC. SCI., is Director of The Stillbirth Association and a member of both the British Association of Social Workers and the Association of Family Therapists. She also helps to train bereavement counselors and family therapists in London, England.

ANDREA MARKS, M.D., is Chief, Division of Adolescent Medicine, Department of Pediatrics, North Shore University Hospital, Manhasset, N.Y. and Assistant Professor of Pediatrics, Cornell Medical College, New York, N.Y.

BARBARA ECK MENNING, R. N., M.S., is founder and director of Resolve, Inc., a national nonprofit organization that offers counseling, support, and referral to infertile couples based in Belmont, Massachussets. She is the author of *Infertility: A Guide for the Childless Couple* and numerous chapters and articles in books and journals.

AMY MILLER-COHEN, PH.D., is co-founder of Pondering Parenthood Workshops and in private practice where she conducts family and marital therapy. She was formerly an Assistant Professor at Brooklyn College, City University of New York and on the staff of Womanschool, New York.

JOAN OFFERMAN-ZUCKERBERG, Ph.D., is founder of Psychological Consultation Service for Parents and Prospective Parents, and in private practice of psychoanalytic psychotherapy. She is Adjunct Assistant Professor of Psychology at Long Island University and a consultant to agencies and obstetricians in the New York metropolitan area.

EDNA ORTOF, PH.D., is a Supervisor and on the faculty of the William Alanson White Institute of Psychoanalysis. She is also Assistant Clinical Professor of Psychology, Department of Psychiatry, Cornell University Medical College; Assistant Attending Psychologist at New York Hospital, Westchester Division; and in private practice.

WILLIAM A. PARKER JR., A.I.A., is Director of the Health Services Planning and Design Program and an Assistant Professor of Architecture at the Graduate School of Architecture and Planning at Columbia University, New York.

JOAN RAPHAEL-LEFF, M.SC., is a clinical and social psychologist and an associate member of both the International Psychoanalytic Association and of the British Psychoanalytic Association. She has been on the Senior Scientific Staff, Medical Research Council, Social Psychiatry Unit, Institute of Psychiatry, London, and has been Senior Psychologist, Children's Department and Adult Out-Patient Department, Malborough Hospital, London, England.

LOUISE SILVERSTEIN, M.A., is a clinical instructor in psychiatry at the State University of New York, Downstate Medical Center, Brooklyn, New York.

JULIE SPAIN, PH.D., was Director of Hoboken Family Planning, Inc., and Senior Psychologist/Clinical Instructor in the Department of Child and Adolescent Psychiatry, Downstate Medical Center in New York. She now consults to DHEW family planning programs, is writing a series of family planning booklets for teenagers, and is in private practice in New York City.

PATSY TURRINI, C.S.W., was an initiator of the Model Mothers' Center, Hicksville, Long Island. She is on the faculty of the Adelphi School of Social Work, and of the Institute for the Training of Psychotherapy. She is in private practice on Long Island.

PHYLLIS URMAN-KLEIN, A.C.S.W., is an Associate in the Department of Psychiatry, Albert Einstein College of Medicine; Chief Social Worker in the Adult Psychiatric Clinic, and a member of the family therapy faculty. She is presently engaged in research on dual career marriages.

GAIL WASSERMAN, PH.D., is a Research Associate in both the Department of Psychiatry, Cornell University Medical College,

New York, and the Department of Pediatrics, College of Physicians and Surgeons, Columbia University, New York. She is a member of the Society for Research in Child Development.

SUE ROSENBERG ZALK, PH.D., is an Associate Professor at Hunter College, City University of New York and on the staff of Eastside Consultation Center/Center for Creative Living. She coauthored *Expectant Fathers* with Sam Bittman. She is actively engaged in research on the psychology of women and is in private practice in New York City.

INTRODUCTION

Barbara L. Blum

Pregnancy and childbirth are major life events, not only for persons who experience them but also for those who, because of conscious or unconscious choices, or because of untreatable physical barriers, do not. Many factors influence our response and adaptation to these events: individual motivations, sociocultural supports and expectations, religious affiliations, and medical procedures are among them. Because of many developments in culture and in medical technology, personal needs and societal attitudes related to pregnancy, childbirth, and parent–infant bonding are changing. These changes have considerable implications for individuals as well as for society as a whole.

Early psychoanalytic theorists (e.g., Freud, Karl Abraham) discussed the role of unconscious motivations in pregnancy and childbirth experiences. Freud (1900), for example, made note of dreams indicating that the wish to have a child often was marked by ambivalence. He found that this ambivalence was sometimes expressed physically in such hysterical symptoms as nausea and vomiting. Further, he observed that dream symbols might announce a pregnancy (e.g., being plagued by vermin; finding milk stains on a blouse) or might specifically refer to giving birth (e.g., rescuing a child from water). Also, Freud (1908) reported women's oral fantasies about conception resulting from eating or swallowing. Perhaps Freud's most famous formulation regarding pregnancy and the unconscious was his theory that a woman's wish to have a child is the result of penis envy (1925).

Although early psychoanalytic references were scattered and incomplete, most of Freud's observations are still pertinent. Thus many contributors to this book (e.g., Miller-Cohen, Ortof, Raphael-Leff, Turrini, and Zuckerberg) discuss ambivalences and unconscious motivations in contemporary pregnancies.

But Freud's penis envy hypothesis has been widely questioned and disputed. Many critics (e.g., Horney, 1967; Millet, 1969) have pointed to the cultural and sexual biases prevalent in the first part of this century as responsible for the development of this concept. Perhaps these same biases also accounted, in part, for the scarcity of discussions of psychological and social factors affecting pregnancy and childbirth during those years. Recent changes in our society have probably helped to create an atmosphere that is more receptive to open discussion of these events. These sociocultural and technological changes also may have created a need for psychological explanations and supports where such need was not felt previously. As science, knowledge, and technology have replaced ritual and superstition, psychological theory has evolved. As women's needs and potentials have been recognized, their traditional roles as primarily childbearers and mothers have been questioned. In short, psychological explorations and explanations of the phenomena of pregnancy and childbirth have developed parallel to a changing society.

Pregnancy and childbirth, as other life transitions, have always been times when conflicts and feelings regarding one's adequacy, fears, hopes, and relationships to past generations arise. Pregnancy, childbirth, and parenting involve major life changes in the woman's body, in interpersonal relationships, in the dynamics of the family, and in social status. Childbirth implies the birth of a life-style as well as of a child; new roles are taken on, old roles are discarded, and social patterns may change. People's ability to cope with the stresses of major life transitions, which is dependent upon their available ego resources as well as upon the sociocultural milieu, results either in psychological growth or in disturbance. In the past, culture and religion provided men and women with elaborate ceremonies, rites, and rituals to mark and to help them cope with the anxieties and conflicts of life transitions. Reik (1946) and Malinowski (1948) discuss couvade* and other such rituals related specifically to pregnancy and childbirth. In our postindustrialized society, while some religious ceremonies remain (e.g., circumcision, baptism), most cultural rituals regarding conception, pregnancy, and childbirth have been discarded. Yet, much of the anxiety persists. In fact, new anxieties and new stresses, resulting from medical, cultural, and technological changes have emerged (e.g., see chapters by Eichholz, Haire, Turrini).

Current psychological theories, such as developmental ego psychology (e.g., Hartmann, 1958), psychosocial theory (e.g., Erikson, 1963), and humanistic psychology (e.g., Maslow, 1968) and many widely read popular books such as Gail Sheehy's *Passages* (1976) and The Boston Women's Health Book Collective's *Our Bodies Our Selves* (1971) have possibly developed in order to replace the psychological support once provided by rituals, and to provide modern men and women with guidelines and a framework in which to experience normal life transitions. These theories, which have influenced contemporary psychological positions regarding pregnancy as a developmental crisis (e.g., Benedek, 1970; Bibring et al., 1961;

---

*Couvade rituals are customs in which, after a child is born, a man takes to his bed, cares for the child, fasts and purifies himself, or engages in magical procedures to protect the child from demons.

Friederich, 1977) also reflect a changing psychological focus: from mental illness, disease, and the abnormal, the emphasis has shifted to mental health, coping, choice, and self-actualization. With this more positive focus, it is likely that common expected psychological experiences in pregnancy and childbirth will be given more attention and study.

Medical advances in the last 50 years also have contributed to an increasing interest in, and awareness of, psychological dimensions of pregnancy and childbirth. Thanks to the development of medical procedures such as ultrasound, amniocentesis, radiography, and fetoscopy, we can now *prenatally* detect many gross developmental or life-threatening abnormalities (e.g. Down's syndrome, Tay-Sachs disease, spina bifida). Because of medical technology and pharmacological breakthroughs, previously unviable fetuses and newborns now survive. Infant and maternal mortality rates have declined significantly. These medical developments have had significant psychological consequences. In the past, because of dangers and deaths, each pregnancy could not provide as much hope, joy, and planning as most pregnancies can promise today. Parental bonding to children was restrained and mourning for deceased children was limited. Superstitions and constraints such as not discussing pregnancy in public, employing euphemisms such as "in a family way," "expecting," "in a delicate condition," and not publicly naming the child until (s)he was born abounded to avoid tempting the hand of fate. With little perceived personal or even medical control over success in pregnancy and birthing, people did not develop the same psychological attachments to pregnancies and infants that they do today. Now, more certain that a pregnancy will result in a live healthy child, we are freer to discuss factors which might influence emotional development during pregnancy and childbirth as well as those which could affect future bonding and relationship to the child.

The development of safe reliable contraceptive techniques and the availability of legal abortions also have affected dramatically the interest in the psychological aspects of pregnancy and childbearing (see Spain, and Ortof in this book for discussions of motivational factors in contraception and abortion). Formerly, procreation could not reliably be separated from sex and sexually active women bore the consequences. Today, women and men alike can actively and consciously choose to separate sex from childbearing. Further, as a result of social pressures to recognize women's sexual needs and desires, women are *psychologically freer* to discuss pregnancy and childbirth openly as aspects of their sexuality.

Industrialization, which has created major changes in the working and living patterns of men and women, also affected attitudes toward pregnancy. In agrarian societies, children were necessary for family and national survival. They provided field labor, income, old age insurance, and social security for their parents; for their countries, they provided national defense. In such societies, womanhood, childbearing, and motherhood were one; childless women were pitied. But in industrialized nations, children are expensive to raise, there is concern about overpopulation, and women are needed in the technological workforce. This has resulted in people becoming more conscious of negative or ambivalent feelings about parenthood. Women are considering role options other than motherhood and men are becoming more aware of their changing roles in the home and in the marketplace.

Today, in many nations, women can and do find gratification in activities other than parenting. Some women choose not to bear children and, perhaps, become involved in full-time work or careers; others, in part as a result of increasing life spans, spend a considerable porportion of their adult lives in activities other than parenting.

The increasing and active participation of women in all aspects of our society, and government legislation for equal status and rights for men and women, has contributed greatly to the increasing recognition of, and positive attitudes toward, women's potentials and needs. As social psychology research indicates, we have a need to maintain consistency, harmony, and congruence between our behavior and attitudes. When behavior changes, therefore, it is likely that attitude change will follow. Perhaps attitudes toward women as primarily child-bearers and childrearers, and condescending attitudes toward women, and even what Reik (1946) and Horney (1967) referred to as male fear and envy of female sexuality and reproductive abilities, will subside and change further as more men and women share tasks of parenting and roles and responsibilities in business and at home.

All of the cultural and medical advances that have been discussed: the evolution of psychological theories, prenatal detection of abnormalities, increased infant survival rates, development of reliable contraception techniques, industrialization, and the changing roles of men and women have contributed to the making of a society where becoming pregnant and giving birth can involve making many conscious as well as unconscious choices. Married career women and their husbands now decide whether or not to have children (Miller-Cohen). Single career women also consider becoming parents (Engelstein et al.) Adolescents (Marks) and older women (Eichholz, Zuckerberg) now have options available regarding becoming and remaining pregnant. Infertile couples can choose to seek psychological counseling as well as medical advice (Menning). Persons already pregnant can choose male or female obstetrician or midwife, and birthing environments in hospitals, birthing centers or at home (Eichholtz, Parker). They may seek professionals using delivery procedures such as the Le Boyer approach (Kliot and Silverstein). Women may seek professional help to understand their body changes (Barry, Zuckerberg) or their special psychologial needs while pregnant (Raphael-Leff). Men too may elect to consider the effects of *their* motivations and needs upon women's pregnancies (Barry & Adler, Zalk) and professionals may consider the effects of their own pregnancies upon their clients or patients (Barbanel).

Decisions during delivery might involve the use of medications, anesthesia, or surgery (Haire). Should the neonate be abnormal or stillborn, decisions including how and what to tell the family need to be made (Fleischman & Fryd, Lewis). Creating conditions conducive to bonding also is of concern to many parents (Wasserman).

Some people elect to leave decisions and choices regarding pregnancy and childbirth to authority figures (e.g., doctors, clergy) and remain passive and dependent. Others question procedures, attitudes and methods, and become active participants in the choices made. The control exerted over pregnancy and childbirth choices probably is representative of the manner in which these persons handle other important life decisions.

In addition to increasing the options available, the changes discussed have resulted in a redefinition of the boundaries of pregnancy and childbirth experiences. One need only observe the avid world interest in the birth of Louise Brown, the first test tube baby, to become aware of the anxieties and hopes that are generated when humankind goes beyond previously established limits. Artificial insemination and test tube babies are current realities; phenomena such as out-of-the-uterus incubation may too become actualities.

The effects of these expanding boundaries of pregnancy and childbirth on the human psyche is very much open to question. With amniocentesis, some abnormalities, as well as the sex of the child, can be detected well within the 24-week legal abortion limit in New York State. Because abnormalities are now an accepted reason for abortion, the range of individual differences in our world, as well as our tolerance for deviation, might change. Population statistics and balances might be affected. Hypothetically, a person might decide to abort a perfect fetus because it is not the desired sex. Merely the possibility of aborting an imperfect or deviant fetus may affect our psyches, and those of our children.

Society will have to make difficult adjustments to these new developments. We will have to decide what, if any, limitations to place on procedures that allow us to tamper with natural selection. And as the needs, attitudes, choices, and issues related to these normal life events, pregnancy and childbirth, become more apparent and even change, continued psychological inquiry and attention will be very important. This is a tremendous responsibility.

All of the contributors to this book are professionals working with people for whom pregnancy, childbirth, and parent–infant bonding are prominent concerns. They explore, from many perspectives, psychological, sociocultural, and medical factors which affect responses to these events. Each, in her or his own manner, has already played a part in expanding the boundaries of our consciousness about psychological aspects of, and needs in, pregnancy, birthing, and bonding.

REFERENCES

Benedek, T. The psychobiology of pregnancy. In E.J. Anthony & T. Benedek (Eds.). *Parenthood: Its psychology and psychopathology.* Boston: Little Brown, 1970.

Bibring, G.L., Dwyer, T.F., Huntington, D.S., & Valenstein, A.F. A study of the psychological process in pregnancy and the earliest mother child relationship. *The Psychoanalytic study of the Child,* 1961, *16,* 6–72.

Boston Women's Health Book Collective. *Our bodies ourselves.* New York: Simon and Schuster, 1971.

Erikson, E. *Childhood and society.* New York: Norton, 1963.

Freud, S. The interpretation of dreams. *The complete psychological works of Sigmund Freud.* Vol. IV and V. London: Hogarth Press, 1900.

Freud, S. On the sexual theories of children. *The complete psychological works of Sigmund Freud,* Vol. IX. London: Hogarth Press, 1908.

Freud, S. Some psychological consequences of anatomical differences between the sexes. *The complete psychological works of Sigmund Freud,* Vol. XIX, London: Hogarth Press, 1925.

Friederich, M. Psychological changes during pregnancy. *Contemporary Ob/ Gyn,* 1977, *9,* 27–34.

Hartmann, H. *Ego psychology and the problem of adaptation.* New York: International Universities Press, 1958.

Horney, K. *Feminine psychology.* New York: Norton, 1967.
Malinowski, B. *Magic, science and religion.* New York: Doubleday, 1948.
Maslow, A. *Toward a psychology of being.* New York: Nostrand, 1968.
Millet, K. *Sexual politics.* New York: Ballantine, 1969.
Reik, T. *Ritual: psychoanalytic studies.* New York: International Universities Press, 1946.
Sheehy, G. *Passages.* New York: Dutton, 1976.

Part I

PSYCHOLOGICAL ISSUES IN BECOMING AND REMAINING PREGNANT

Many factors, including health, marital status, age, relationships with peers, stage of psychosocial development, and intrapsychic needs and conflicts regarding love, parenting, sexuality, and anger contribute to behaviors resulting in pregnancy. One theme in this section is that, for most modern women and men, becoming pregnant can be a choice, one motivated by unconscious as well as by conscious needs and fantasies. The contributors to this section explore how and why choices resulting in either planned or unplanned pregnancies are made. For women who cannot conceive, or who miscarry or choose abortion, the effects of losing both the child and also the fantasies associated with pregnancy and parenthood are discussed.

chapter 1

PSYCHOLOGICAL ISSUES IN INFERTILITY

Barbara Eck Menning

When Rachel saw that she bore Jacob no children . . .
she said to Jacob, "Give me children or I die!"

Genesis 30:1

The control over unwanted pregnancy has increased steadily in America since World War II. The condom and foam of the prewar generations gave way to the more reliable diaphragm and then to the birth control pill and IUD. Couples can now engage in active and spontaneous sexual relations secure in the knowledge that their birth control method approaches 98 percent in effectiveness. Many Americans now plan their families as meticulously as they do their education, field of endeavor, living situation and major financial investments—measuring all factors and waiting until the moment for starting a family is exactly right:

Six years ago my husband and I got married. We knew that children would definitely be a part of our life. The question was not IF, but WHEN. We waited several years to let me use my college degree, to buy a house, and to establish a good foundation before we brought children into the world. . . .

I sit here, six years later. I have a wonderful husband, established roots, the house of my dreams, years of teaching experience. But the children we had longed for are denied us.

For one out of every six couples of childbearing age, fertility is not a force that can be turned on at will. Infertility, the inability to achieve pregnancy after a year of regular sexual relations, or the inability to carry pregnancy to a live birth, will be experienced by 15 percent of the population of childbearing age. A recent report from the U.S. Census Bureau (estimates and projections based on July 1, 1978) tells us that there are now 220 million Americans. Because of a baby boom in the postwar 1940s and 1950s, there are about 60 million people, or 30 percent of our total population between the ages of 22 and 40 years of age. If we apply the accepted rate of infertility to this number, we reach a number in excess of 10 million who may, at some time, be unable to achieve or carry pregnancy. Menning (1977) states that of this number about 40 percent have an infertility problem solely related to the female; 40 percent have a problem solely related to the male; and the remaining 20 percent have a problem which either affects both members of the couple, or is of unknown origin.

Fortunately, medical investigation and treatment has made great strides in helping to cure infertility in recent years. It is now estimated that at least half of all infertility can be diagnosed and treated by either medical or surgical means. To achieve this excellent rate of success, it is imperative that infertile couples find a physician who has special expertise and interest in the area of infertility. Some of the most reknowned specialists claim cure rates in excess of 60 to 70 percent; however, diagnosis and treatment are not without physical, emotional, and financial expenditure, sometimes adding up to many years of effort and numerous expert opinions before the longed for pregnancy results.

For approximately five million Americans, conceiving and

carrying a pregnancy to a live birth will prove impossible. This population represents one of the most invisible and therefore neglected minority groups in our country. They suffer neither a medical illness, in most cases, nor a mental illness. They have what some have termed a social condition, that of involuntary childlessness. This condition exacts a heavy toll on their physical and psychological well-being, and on the quality of their life.

Since 1973 I have worked as a counselor of infertile people. As founder and Director of RESOLVE, a national, nonprofit organization that deals solely with the needs of infertile couples, I have become aware of the particular issues that infertility represents to most men and women. During the past six years I have done extensive telephone counseling, led support groups (for both women and couples), edited a newsletter, and more recently done individual and couple crisis intervention counseling.

There is growing proof that the infertility rate is on the rise in this country and around the world. There are a number of sociological and medical factors involved. One of the most important is the trend toward delaying marriage and child-bearing into the years after 30. While this has sound economic and emotional rationale, it is known that both women and men are maximally fertile in their mid-20s, and that fertility in women falls off rapidly in the years after 30. Also, some major causes of infertility in women, such as endometriosis, are much more prevalent in the older woman. Other factors increasing the infertility rate are the recent rise in venereal disease, prolonged use or misuse of certain birth control methods (notably the pill and IUD), and exposure of both men and women to toxins, drugs, and environmental conditions which may put them at risk for future fertility. A dramatic example of the last category is DES daughters and sons, who are just now entering the childbearing years and who have been found to have an increased incidence of reproductive abnormalities and infertility. It is estimated that between 1940 and 1970 DES was prescribed for up to 6 million women. The United States Department of Health, Education, and Welfare estimates that half of those are unaware of their exposure.

There has probably never been a more difficult time to be infertile. At the same time that the infertility rate is increasing, the alternative of adoption of a healthy local infant has never been more difficult. While it appears that as many out-of-wedlock pregnancies are occurring as ever before, it is also true that about 90 percent of single mothers retain their babies instead of surrendering them for adoption. A couple wishing to adopt a local infant may face a wait of from 3 to 5 years at most metropolitan adoption agencies. Increasing numbers of couples are exploring adoption from international sources, or are forced to reconcile themselves to a life without children. Those with male infertility problems are turning to artificial insemination by donor in record numbers. All of these latter options force the couple to face adjustments and issues which may be as difficult as the original problem of infertility. There are no longer any easy answers.

THE FEELINGS OF THE INFERTILE COUPLE

Infertility is a complex life crisis which evokes many feelings. Some feelings are rational, based on the very real and difficult events of the social and medical situation. Others may be more irrational, based in part upon myths and superstitions, or on childlike magical thinking. The feelings vary in order and intensity, but it has been my experience as an infertility couselor that most people face a similar syndrome of feelings as they attempt to work through infertility. The order which I have most often observed, and which is quite logical, will be described here. The anecdotal material quoted throughout this chapter comes from actual case histories.

Surprise

The first reaction most people have to news of infertility is one of total shock and surprise. Most couples in their child-bearing years are used to thinking in terms of *prevention* of pregnancy. They naturally assume that they could have children if and when they desire them. It is ironic that most couples discover their infertility after having used some form of birth control, sometimes for many years. The discovery of an infertility problem is felt most keenly by those who are highly achievement oriented, and who believe themselves capable of surmounting any obstacle if only enough effort and will are exerted.

Denial

"This can't happen to me!" is often the reaction to infertility, especially if the initial tests reveal an absolute and untreatable problem in either partner. Denial serves a purpose. It allows the mind and body to adjust at their own rate to an overwhelming situation. Denial is only dangerous when it becomes a long-term or permanent coping mechanism. I have seen chronically depressed women who staunchly maintain that they never *really* wanted a family and both men and women who refused to apply the label "infertile" to themselves in spite of 5 or 10 years of involuntary childlessness. People who need this level of defense are usually in need of psychotherapy of some duration.

Anger

When a couple enter into an infertility investigation and attempted treatment, they surrender much of their control over their bodies. Even in the best doctor–patient relationship, frustration, helplessness, and embarrassment may be present. Anger is a predictable response to loss of control. The anger may be quite rational and focused on real and correctly perceived insults, such as social pressuring from family and friends to "produce," and the pain and inconvenience of the tests and treatments. Sometimes the anger is of a more irrational nature, projected onto targets such as the doctor or the marriage partner, or even onto social issues such as Pro-Choice abortion advocates, or people who "breed like rabbits." This irrational anger is usually a front for a more primary feeling, such as intense loss and grief, which cannot yet be acknowledged. Whatever the source or the type of anger, it is very necessary that the person be able to ventilate it. Anger tends to dissipate in the telling (and retelling) of the indignities producing it. This can be done without detriment to the angry person or others in a milieu such as a peer support group.

Isolation

It is common for an infertile couple to state that they are the *only* people they know who cannot achieve a pregnancy. Infertility is a difficult subject for most people to discuss. It is very personal and inherently sexual. Couples may keep their infertility a secret because they do not wish to be objects of pity, or fear receiving unsolicited adivice, such as, "relax!" or "Why don't you take a second honeymoon?!" Secrecy may have several negative effects. It usually increases the pressuring and needling from family and friends about the couples' plans to start a family. More important, it cuts the couple off from potential sources of comfort and support in a time of great stress. In extreme cases, infertile couples may be so sensitized to the sight of pregnant women or children that they withdraw from any social situation which might produce such a contact. This may even involve a change of work or living situation.

Isolation may occur between the members of a couple as well. The woman may despair over her husband's inability to empathize with her feelings about menstruation, her fixation on her basal temperature chart around ovulation time, or her nervous hopes if a period goes overdue. The man may find it impossible to share his anxiety over being "counted and scored" in semen analysis, or having to perform sex on demand whether he feels like it or not. The result may be a breakdown in communication and a loss of pleasure in the sexual relationship. Marital stress and tension over sex are so commonly present in certain phases of infertility that in my counseling I am amazed if I do not discover them. Since the couple often have no others to validate their feelings, they may presume that not only are they infertile, but that their marriage and sex life are in jeopardy. It is always a relief when infertile couples find each other and hear that they share the same frustrations and concerns. One of the most helpful ways to ease the isolation of infertility is to help couples find each other and join in a support group experience.

Guilt

Another reason for the secrecy that so often surrounds infertility is the presence of guilt. People seem to need to construct a cause-and-effect relationship for events that happen to them. The infertile couple review their mutual and individual histories and search for a guilty deed for which they are being punished. Some of the common guilt producers I have seen in my counseling are premarital sex, use of birth control, a previous abortion; venereal disease: extramarital sex or interest, masturbation, homosexual thoughts or acts, and even sexual pleasure itself. Once the guilty deed is discovered, the infertile person may go to great lengths to atone and achieve forgiveness. Atoning may take any form, from religious acts, to personal denial, to working in painful areas such as counseling of unwed mothers or teaching other people's children. Guilt and atonement appear to have no relationship to the educational level of the person. Some of the most sophisticated people I have counseled have applied a mystical belief in "God's punishment" to their own infertility, even in the absence of belief in a religion.

Certainly the teachings of the Old Testament and folklore from early civilization play into seeing the infertile person (particularly the woman) as fallen from grace or being punished by higher powers. People who have poor self-esteem seem particularly vulnerable to guilty thoughts about infertility. Believing in their hearts that they really do not deserve a pregnancy and child, they may keep their infertility very secret for fear it might be discovered how "bad" they really are.

Grief

Without question, the most compelling feeling of conclusive infertility is grief. This state may be preceded by a period of depression, as the final throes of testing or treatment are pursued to no avail. Once all hope for pregnancy and live birth is abandoned, the appropriate and necessary response should be grieving. It is a strange and puzzling kind of grief, involving the loss of a potential, not of an actual life. One woman I counseled described it in these words:[1]

> Death. Death of a lot of things. It is the end of the Bowes' family and the Bowes family name. It dies with us because of me. My husband is the last of the male children in his family. Death before life . . . before we even knew our child, because he never existed. The hardest part of this kind of death is that it is the death of a dream. There are no solid memories, no pictures, no things to remember. You can't remember your child's blond hair, or brown eyes, or his favorite toys or the way he laughed, or the way it felt to be pregnant with him. He never existed.

Society has elaborate rituals to comfort the bereaved in death (See Lazare [1976] for an excellent discussion of the psychology of bereavement.) Infertility is different; there is no funeral, no wake, no grave to lay flowers on. Family and friends may never even know. The infertile couple often come to this point of grief

[1]The real name has been changed to preserve confidentiality.

alone. Stillbirth or miscarriage, while very tragic, is more often perceived as an actual death. Family and friends are more often aware of the loss and offer solace and support.

Infertility which is conclusive represents many losses: the loss of children; the loss of genetic continuity; the loss of fertility, and all that fertility means to attitudes toward sexuality; and the loss of the pregnancy experience itself. For each individual, some aspects of loss are keener than others. When grieving over infertility does take place, it is often quite focused and specific. Failure or inability to grieve over infertility is the most common problem I have encountered when dealing with infertile clientele.

There are some very logical reasons why grief may fail. *There may be no recognized loss.* Because infertility represents the loss of a potential not actual object, the couple may not realize that they are entitled to grieve. This may be unwittingly abetted by suggestions from the doctor at the moment of conclusion that "they can always adopt" which send the couple immediately to the search for an alternative.

A second reason is that *the loss may be seen as "socially unspeakable."* Because both male and female infertility are loaded with sexual overtones and possibly guilt feelings, family and friends may feel it is not appropriate to speak of the loss or offer solace. One or both members of the couple may forbid the mention of the subject thereby precluding any progress toward grief and resolution.

A third reason for failure to grieve may be uncertainty over the loss. In a certain percentage of infertility cases, a conclusive diagnosis is never reached. There *could* be a spontaneous pregnancy in any cycle. The couple *could* seek yet another expert opinion. The moment for grieving is elusive, the couple hold back their grief for a moment of certainty. Some have likened this state of limbo to being similar to having a loved one "missing in action" in war. Possible loss is not actual loss. In some cases a conclusion is never experienced until the woman completes her menopause.

A fourth reason for failure to grieve may be absence of a social support system. Grieving is intense and painful. There may be great reluctance to give in to the feelings without the reassuring presence of family and friends to give comfort. It is a fact that 30 percent of our population in America moves every year. We are increasingly a society that is nuclear and without roots. When the need to grieve arises, infertile people may find themselves far away from the loved ones they need for comfort. Those who find themselves isolated in this way often seek out the help of a therapist, counselor, or support group.

As painful as initial griefwork may be—accompanied by weeping, and sobbing, and physical symptoms such as loss of appetite, exhaustion, choking, or tightness in the throat—it does run a predictable course and it does end. It is helpful to point this out to the person who is afraid to give in to the feelings. Assisting a person or couple through griefwork is a most rewarding experience. As a "grief facilitator," I have often seen the cleansing and restorative powers of a good grief.

Resolution

The desired goal of any crisis, including infertility, is its successful resolution. The process of resolution requires that each of the difficult feelings detailed here be discovered, worked through, and overcome. Feelings are never laid away forever; they may be activated by special reminders, such as anniversaries of losses, or by new and different crises. But the feelings are never as difficult or overwhelming as they were. Reactivation is usually brief and can be accepted by the person rather philosophically.

People I have counseled about infertility describe the state of resolution in some of the following ways: there is a return of energy, perhaps even a surge of zest and well-being; a sense of perspective emerges which puts infertility in its proper place in life; a sense of optimism and faith returns; a sense of humor returns and some of the past absurdities may even become grist for a good story. The concepts of sexuality, self image, and self-esteem are reworked to become disconnected from child-bearing, but nevertheless wholesome and complete. Plans for the future are begun again, building a way around the obstacle of infertility. The couple are ready to act with confidence in selecting an alternative life plan (such as adoption). Once resolution is achieved, the couple is ready to get on with their lives.

SOME AREAS OF SPECIAL CONCERN

It is beyond the scope of this chapter to undertake an in-depth discussion of the special situations which raise troublesome issues for infertile couples. Infertility is a complex life crisis. It rarely proceeds as ideally as described, from discovery of a problem, working through feelings to resolution, and developing an alternative plan for building a family. Four situations were selected to represent some of the more convoluted issues involved in infertility. Following, I will discuss briefly the couple who experience miscarriage or stillbirth; the "normal infertile" couple; the couple who choose to have a child by donor insemination; and the couple who conceive after years of effort. For a more detailed discussion of these subjects, the reader is invited to consult the references at the end of this chapter.

Miscarriage and Stillbirth

One aspect of infertility concerns itself not with the inability of a couple to achieve a pregnancy, but with problems that result in loss of the pregnancy before a live birth. Miscarriage[2] is a more common occurrence than many people realize. It is estimated that one in six pregnancies ends this way. Seventy-five percent of all miscarriages occur in the first trimester and

[2]The term *miscarriage* is used instead of the more medically correct term *spontaneous abortion*, to avoid confusion with therapeutic abortion.

are due to unavoidable and untreatable problems. These random mistakes of nature rarely repeat themselves in the child-bearing years of normal couples. Infertile couples may be defined as those who have repeated miscarriages, probably due to some other structural or hormonal problem. It also appears that couples who have had great difficulty in conceiving are at greater risk. It is thought that they run a 40 percent risk of miscarriage, often due to the very problems which made them have trouble conceiving.

Medically, a miscarriage is a potentially dangerous, even life-threatening situation. When emotional aspects are added to the physical trauma, this may be seen as a life event of critical importance. The following quote is from *Our Bodies Ourselves* (1976):

> We did not understand what was happening and why . . . Did this mean something was wrong with one of us? Did this mean we could NEVER have children? Had I done something wrong during the early months to cause this miscarriage? We were so frightened by the amount and look of what was pouring out of me . . . It wasn't bad enough that we were losing our baby, but in the midst of all that pain, we had to stay strong enough to deal with all that blood.(p. 317)

Miscarriage is almost always totally unexpected. It may be over with in a matter of minutes in early pregnancy, or it may drag on for days or even weeks. Occasionally medical intervention is successful in preventing loss of pregnancy. The couple going through such heroics may experience alternate states of hope and despair as they wait to see their fate. Most often the onset of bleeding and cramping will continue through to complete expulsion of the fetus.

There are a number of issues unique to the experience of miscarriage. One of the most troublesome is the practice of many hospitals of admitting the patient who threatens to miscarry into the obstetric unit. There she may be in close proximity with laboring and newly delivered patients and also the newborn nursery. Hospitals justify this policy by explaining that miscarriage is not a routine gynecologic event and needs to be managed in the cleaner obstetric area where the delivery room is available for surgical intervention. The emotional effect on the couple, however, may be profound. One woman said:

> Seeing a basinet in the delivery room as I was being prepared for a D & C after my miscarriage really blew my mind. I started screaming, "Get that thing out of there—there IS NO BABY!" At that point they sedated me. When I woke up I was in the recovery room next to a newly delivered woman. She asked me, "Did you have a boy or a girl?

The couple who have experienced a miscarriage should, at the very least, be screened from laboring and newly delivered patients. A special indicator should be posted on the door so that hospital staff are aware of the situation. The husband should not be treated as a "visitor" but allowed unlimited access to his wife. Privacy from all but a few caretenders will facilitate the couple in expressing their grief.

The need for grieving after a miscarriage, especially for the couple who have longed for a child, is obvious. Unfortunately, many hospital personnel are uncomfortable with this basic, human emotion. Grieving may be seen by them as "suffering" or disturbing to the welfare of other patients. It is all too common for doctors to prescribe sedation, tranquilizers or even mood-elevating drugs so that no one need be "upset." Probably the best management of the grieving couple is the earliest possible discharge home, where both griefwork and recovery can take place unimpeded.

The reaction of significant others to news of a miscarriage is usually one of abbreviated support (one client termed it a "minideath") and assurances of successful pregnancy in the near future. It has been my experience, that if well-meaning family and friends say anything at all, it is usually the wrong thing. "It's a blessing. The baby wouldn't have been normal. . . ." "Next year this time you'll be up to your elbows in diapers!" Such platitudes and assurances are not only medically unsound, they invalidate the couples' right to grieve for *this* particular loss.

I have witnessed a few cases where couples endured five or six or more miscarriages before giving up hope. They received news of each subsequent pregnancy with dread instead of joy. They kept the pregnancy secret for fear of raising anyone's hopes, and they practiced denial heavily themselves to prevent their own nervous hopes from mounting with each passing week. The emotional toll in such cases is exhausting. I have known several couples who finally chose sterilization in preference to any more attempts at pregnancy.

Stillbirth is technically the loss of a baby which has reached sufficient gestation to be viable outside the womb (usually after 28 weeks). It is a much less common occurrence and usually not a recurring event. There are several possible situations, each fraught with its own pain and turmoil. There may be a cessation of fetal life, where the couple are admitted to the hospital knowing their baby is dead before delivery. There may be a viable baby who expires in the labor or delivery process, or due to congenital abnormalities at birth when separated from its placental blood supply. In these cases the death is not anticipated. And finally there may be a crisis for both mother and child, such as premature separation of the placenta, where bleeding may be profuse and the oxygenation of the baby is interrupted. This latter example is a life-threatening situation and the emotional issues become secondary to the medical emergency.

Whatever the circumstance, several common issues arise. The couple will inevitably be admitted to the labor and delivery area and afterward to the postpartum unit. Screening and privacy from normally laboring and delivering patients and in the recovery phase is paramount. If the baby is known to be dead, delivery by the least hazardous means to the woman and attendance of the husband or another person to comfort is recommended. It appears to be important to the grieving process for the couple to be able to view and handle the body of the baby. This should be offered if requested and suggested sensitively if not requested. Since autopsy is often done in these circumstances, it is best for the couple to view the body before it is sent to pathology. The woman who has had a stillbirth is in a postpartum state of recovery, as well as a state of grieving. She will have all the needs of the usual postpartum patient in addition to her emotional needs. Sensitive caretending and nurturance from hospital staff plus unlimited access to her husband will facilitate recovery.

The couple who have been through a miscarriage or stillbirth need to know "why." They may fantasize that they did something wrong that resulted in this event. If anything of medical value can be discovered by pathology, especially if it has bearing on future pregnancies, this should by all means be sought and shared.

The "Normal Infertile" Couple

For approximately 10 percent of couples with infertility, no physical or metabolic problem is ever found to account for the fact that they do not conceive. The term "normal infertile" has been applied to this population, though, in the words of Kistner (1973), "The so-called normal infertile couple obviously is not normal or they would not have an infertility problem."

Because there is no physical finding, in spite of second, third, or more expert opinions the couple with this problem often fall prey to suggestions that the problem may be "all in their heads." The visible signs of anxiety, depression, and frustration they manifest as a result of their unending battle, may be mistaken for the cause instead of the effect of the problem. Suggestions from family and friends are made to "relax!" The woman is advised to quit her job (if she is working) or to seek employment (if she is sitting at home in despair). These gratuitous psychiatric offerings can be excused from lay persons, but the truth is that they come too often from the physician and helping professionals as well. Somewhere, etched in early psychoanalytic thought, is the presumption that if a couple have no physical pathology to account for infertility, then they must have some mental pathology. When I hear this suggestion, I am reminded of the words of an infertile friend and colleague, herself a psychiatrist, when a doctor tried to tell her to "relax." She retorted "It so happens I come from a long line of *fertile* female neurotics!"

One of the most compelling issues for the "normal infertile" couple is that they can never quite give up hope of a pregnancy, even though they may make attempts to put infertility out of mind and go on to adopt their family. Each cycle could be the one—each menstruation proves that it was not. Since there is no definite answer, the couple faced with this problem have no clear signal to grieve. I have seen protracted depressive states in such women and men. The ability to enter into griefwork requires acknowledging a loss, and there is no loss. It is my presumption that such couples may experience their final end to hoping only when menopause heralds the end to the woman's "fertile years." I would expect menopause to be more difficult and laden with issues for such couples for this reason. My own experience with people over the age of 45 is, as yet, limited.

Some couples cannot face a life of ceaseless hoping and choose to take active control over their situation by practicing birth control or having sterilization. I believe a strong case can be made for either solution, as it allows the couple to designate an end to hoping, to experience their loss, and to move on to an alternative.

The normal infertile couple have exaggerated emotional needs caused by the cycles of hope and despair they endure. They are particularly vulnerable to exploitation by fads, quackery, and expensive claims for cure. Couples resort to megavitamins, acupuncture, herbal remedies, hypnosis, astrology, faith healers, macrobiotic diets, and the like in the hope of a "cure." The spontaneous cure rate of these couples approaches about 5 percent and probably accounts for the occasional pregnancy which results after such measures have been tried.

The Couple Who Choose Donor Insemination

When infertility rests solely with the male partner, artificial insemination by donor is one possible alternative. Donor insemination has seen an enormous increase in popularity and availability in the last decade. While statistics are hard to verify, it is estimated that at least 10,000 babies are conceived by this technique annually in America. The increasing popularity may be due, in part, to the decreasing supply of healthy young adoptable infants, and also to the increasing acceptability of donor insemination as a medical service. One clinic in the Boston area currently has a 1-year waiting list of people waiting to enter its donor insemination program. This trend is being reflected around the country.

Because of the increasing demand for this alternative, I have seen an increasing number of clients, both in private counseling and in support groups, who wish to work through the issues surrounding donor insemination. I feel this alternative offers an excellent solution for the well screened and counseled couple, as it provides both the longed-for child and also the pregnancy experience. It is disturbing to note that many doctors suggest donor insemination in a casual manner, in the absence of proper screening and counseling. I feel strongly that donor insemination should be considered as an alternative to infertility, not as a treatment. The feelings of both partners, including grief, need to be elaborated before they are ready to take this step.

There are several predominate issues that couples considering donor insemination need to work through. One of the first is their moral, ethical, and philosophical acceptance of the procedure. The Roman Catholic church still views donor insemination as "adultery" and a child so conceived as "illegitimate." People of all religious persuasions have to wrestle with their conscience before coming to complete acceptance of this means to having children. While the counselor cannot offer an opinion about acceptability for a given couple, he or she can often play the objective and nonjudgmental referee in the debate the couple have with each other. Ultimately, the couple must come to a unanimous decision on their own, as it is they who must live with the consequences.

Many women feel "selfish" that they will be achieving a pregnancy without the genetic contribution of the husband. This loss of genetic continuity is an important factor for the husband to discuss and to accept. No matter how well the donor is matched to the husband, this loss is real and needs to be grieved. Some doctors who are apparently uncomfortable with donor insemination, play into "pretending" by mixing donor and husband semen, or by suggesting that the couple have sexual relations immediately after each insemination. I feel this is very unhealthy and should be avoided. Many husbands participate in the insemination process in other ways, however. They may be physically present during the procedure, and participate fully in the prenatal period, attending childbirth classes and facilitating labor and delivery, just as any other husband would. I strongly encourage full participation of this kind. For the couple who have settled the genetic loss, nothing else need be sacrificed in the donor insemination experience.

Both husband and wife may have exaggerated fears as the time of delivery approaches. One common fear is that a mistake in selection of donor may have been made, resulting in a baby of totally incongruous racial or physical appearance. This fear is the subject of dreams, fantasies, and general anxiety. There may also be more subtle fears regarding the baby's health, intelligence, and attractiveness. Very little information is shared about the donor to preserve anonymity. A great deal of faith must be placed in the hands of the doctor or clinic doing the screening and selecting of donors. This is a sacred trust which no facility offering donor insemination should take lightly. I have noted that couples returning for a second or third pregnancy by donor insemination are much more relaxed and unconcerned about the quality of selection and less fearful of mistakes. Many couples are so delighted with the outcome of the first pregnancy that they request the same donor again, if it is possible.

One of the most difficult issues surrounding donor insemination is the issue of confidentiality. Most doctors recommend that the couple keep the procedure secret between them, since in all but a few states, there is no legal definition of the rights of the child born of donor insemination. Secrecy also protects the couple from the remarks and reactions of society and friends, and from the possibility that the child might discover its origins in a less than desirable way. Every couple I have counseled has struggled with the question of whether or not to tell their child about its manner of conception. Couples often see this question as directly determining whether or not they will share information with close friends and family at the outset. Confidentiality has been hotly debated in support groups I have led. There seems no right or wrong. Again it amounts to the couple doing what they can comfortably live with. One remark made frequently is "you can always decide to tell, but, you cannot untell." This leads most couples to be very discreet in the beginning. One of the obvious tradeoffs in choosing secrecy is that the couple cut themselves off from sources of support. The confidentiality of a support group or counselor is of great benefit here. Even those couples who are very candid and certain that they want their child or children to know about his or her origins cannot agree at all on the right age to share this information or the way to impart the story. Donor insemination is clearly different than adoption, in that it is too sophisticated a subject to be shared when the child first inquires about where babies come from.

The Couple Who Finally Conceive

One final area of special concern is reserved for the couple who have been infertile for many years, then, by medical or spontaneous means, find themselves finally pregnant. Don't they live happily ever after? Quite to the contrary, such couples may have some of the biggest adjustments and disappointments of their life ahead.

When pregnancy and parenting evade a couple for a long time, the experiences tend to become highly idealized and romanticized. Pregnancy is thought of as a time of blooming and glowing. Delivery is thought of as well controlled laboring, and a magnificent birth complete with LeBoyer method or father taking home movies. Breastfeeding is envisioned as a Madonna and child painting of serenity and fulfillment. Parenting? Well, parenting should be a breeze for a couple who have prepared and longed for so many years.

Enter reality:

> Each day of my pregnancy I was plagued with nausea. Never was there a day better than a constant vomitous feeling in my gut. I did not feel I had the privilege of complaining. I had even said to friends that I'd gladly be sick every day of a pregnancy to have a baby! I was totally miserable. Ironically, the only way to relieve the churnings and to fight my anxieties was by eating. Sixty pounds of weight gain attest to their magnitude.

Pregnancy, especially in the woman over 35 is often accompanied by physical distress. Labor and delivery is almost invariably more protracted and difficult than for the younger woman. The cesarean-section rate among formerly infertile women carrying a first pregnancy after 35 is over 25 percent. Breastfeeding may turn out to be a fatiguing and uncomfortable experience for the older woman. Any of these realities might be taken in stride by a couple who knew they would be able to have another pregnancy, or who had not spent years idealizing this state. But there are high stakes riding on pregnancy and parenting for the formerly infertile couple. As a couple already sensitized to loss of control, any of the above problems may hook into their old sense of "failure." In addition, the couple often feel thay have no right to complain. After all, this is their "miracle child" coming into the world.

A number of couples express disappointment when they first view their longed-for baby. As one woman put it, "Is *this* all we get after 7 years of trying?" Of course, love and bonding with a baby must grow and develop over time, for the formerly infertile as well as anyone else. But the difference is in the couple's expectations of an instant love and a perfect relationship. If the child proves to be colicky, or inclined toward purple rages instead of sweet smiles, or if the child is less than perfect and beautiful, the couple may again feel vulnerable to their old sense of failure. The formerly infertile are in a sense "set up," since no pregnancy or parenting experience can live up to their expectations. No mere newborn is able to make up for years of trial and anguish. In fact, the baby is not able to *give* anything to them at all. It is just going to make necessary demands on their energies and time for many months, without the slightest consideration of their needs.

Many formerly infertile women cannot leave a child with a baby sitter or return to their career without intense feelings of guilt. To have longed for a child for years and then surrender it to someone else's care seems hypocrisy. If this child is the only one the couple can ever conceive, the potential for overprotection is great. The child is literally irreplaceable. The parents may have exaggerated needs for the child to conform to their standards and achieve their hopes and dreams.

On the positive side, the couple who conceive after a great deal of time and effort usually bring years of maturity and stability to the parenting situation. There is no question that their child is loved and appreciated, which cannot help but benefit the child's own self-esteem.

MEETING THE NEEDS OF INFERTILE COUPLES

I would like to conclude this chapter by making a special appeal to professionals in mental health and related fields to appreciate the special needs of the infertile couple. In being denied a pregnancy and parenting experience when they truly desire it, they are faced with a life crisis of major proportions. As with any crisis, the couple will find their usual coping mechanisms fail to solve the problem and a period of disequilibrium will result. As we have learned, crisis will push to resolution within a relatively short period of time, with or without intervention. The danger is always that resolution will leave a couple in a less functional, unhealthy state. It is the goal of the person who counsels infertile couples to help them resolve the crisis positively, and to develop new insights and strengths as a result.

One organization which mental health professionals should be aware of is RESOLVE. This national, nonprofit organization was started in 1973 and has as its goals offering counseling, referral, and support to infertile couples. Counseling may be brief and information given by telephone, or may consist of crisis intervention counseling with a trained professional. Referral is made to the best possible source of medical help, as well as to alternative resources such as adoption agencies or donor insemination services. Support is offered largely through the format of peer support groups, which are time limited and led by a trained professional. At this writing, RESOLVE has chapters in 27 cities and publishes a bimonthly newsletter and other helpful information. Through RESOLVE, infertile couples are able to receive support and meet with others who share their experience and concerns.

The infertile couple who so earnestly desire a family deserve respect and attention. They should be seen as having a legitimate health problem which has attendant emotional issues and overtones. Though they are rarely physically "ill" and do not usually find themselves incapable of performing their work and living functions, this very neglected population of some 10 million suffers an enormous toll in the quality of their life. Mental health professionals must be aware of the special feelings and issues of the infertile couple.

REFERENCES

Kistner, R. The infertile woman. *American Journal of Nursing,* 1973, *73,* (11), 1937–1943.

Menning, B. *Infertility: A guide for the childless couple.* Englewood, N.J.: Prentice-Hall, 1977.

Boston Women's Health Book Collective. *Our bodies: ourselves, 2nd ed.* New York: Simon and Schuster, 1976.

Lazare, A. *Community mental health and target populations.* Englewood Cliffs, N.J.: Prentice-Hall, 1976.

BIBLIOGRAPHY

Amelar, R. D., & Dubin, L. Male infertility. *Urology.* 1973, 1–30.

Beck, W. A. A critical look at the legal, ethical, and technical aspects of artificial insemination. *Fertility and Sterility,* 1976, *27,* 1.

Behrman, S. J., & Kistner, R. *Progess in infertility.* Boston: Little Brown, 1975.

Harvey, A. How couples feel about donor insemination. *Contemporary Ob/ Gyn,* 1977, *9,* 93–97.

MacNamera, J. *The adoption advisor.* New York: Hawthorne Books, 1975.

Mazor, M. (ed.) *Medical and psychiatric aspects of infertility.* New York: Human Sciences, (in press).

Mazor, M. The problem of infertility. In M. Notman, & C. Nadelson (Eds.), *The woman patient, Vol. I.* New York: Plenum Press, 1978.

Menning, B. Counseling infertile couples. *Contemporary Ob/Gyn,* 1977, *13,* 101–108.

Menning, B. The infertile couple: A plea for advocacy. *Child Welfare,* 1975, *54,* (6), 454–460.

chapter 2

PSYCHOLOGICAL ASPECTS OF ABORTION

Edna Ortof

In July 1970, the New York State Legislature passed the nation's first law allowing abortion up to 24 weeks of pregnancy. In January 1973, 2–1/2 years later, the Supreme Court ruled to legalize abortion throughout the United States during the first 3 months of pregnancy. In establishing the right of privacy in this matter, it left the choice of abortion a matter for the pregnant woman and her conscience. The court pointed to various detriments the state would impose upon the pregnant woman if the choice of abortion was denied her, such as the stigma of unwed motherhood, the physical and mental stress of additional offspring, the psychological distress of having an unwanted child, and the possible medically diagnosible harm, even in early pregnancy.

With the new laws, the acute anxiety associated with how to go about terminating an unwanted pregnancy was removed. However, the legalization of abortion has not done away with the psychological trauma abortion sometimes causes. The new laws permit the psychological consequences of an abortion to be separated from the panic associated with how to go about obtaining one. These feelings of panic, and the subsequent relief experienced when the abortion was obtained and all went well, often masked other emotional reactions associated with being pregnant, the decision to terminate a pregnancy, and the loss of a pregnancy.

Recently, I was asked if getting an abortion was now as simple as having a tooth pulled. My answer was that both procedures could cause distress. Any of life's circumstances have the potential for generating strong emotional reactions, including abortion or giving birth. That abortion sometimes causes psychological stress should not, therefore, be used as a reason to legislate it away. The constitutional right to abortion is an issue that must be dealt with separately from the psychological stresses of abortion.

Women who cannot or do not want to have a child become pregnant for a variety of conscious and unconscious reasons. Some carry through with the pregnancy giving the child up for adoption. Usually in such cases the idea of abortion conflicts with basic philosophical or religious beliefs. Where the fetus is valued as a life, and abortion equated with murder, adoption is a more viable alternative to enduring guilt.

For women who choose abortion, the weight of evidence suggests that most express relief at their decision regardless of ambivalent feelings, states of guilt, or depression. For many, these uncomfortable feelings are transient, particularly if the abortion is performed early in the pregnancy. Some women, however, have profound emotional reactions to abortion and the effects are long-lasting. Hopes and fantasies are activated, even though the pregnancy is unwanted. Reported dreams during this period tend to actively reflect these fantasies, conflicts, and anxieties.

In my practice, I have worked with a number of women who have had abortions, either during their treatment or sometime prior to it. Their various feelings bracketing the time of the abortion were observed and worked through. The complicated motivations in becoming pregnant were explored. Characterological similarities in women who had unwanted pregnancies were noted. Several of these cases and related dreams will be presented and discussed.

CASE 1

A 21-year-old single college student living with her father, became pregnant by the young man she was seeing regularly. She had been taking oral contraceptives but stopped because she thought they made her depressed. She thinks she became pregnant during her "safe" period when the couple took chances, and was about 15 weeks pregnant when I saw her and her lover for an emergency consultation.

The patient had just seen a gynecologist for the first time, postponing an earlier visit because of her ambivalence over abortion. While she consciously did not want a child, nor was she in a position to care for one, she was under considerable pressure to carry through with the pregnancy. Her lover felt that he had a biological right to the child and begged her not to have an abortion. His harassment created enormous guilt in the patient, making her feel that she was destroying a part of him in terminating the pregnancy. The patient did not want to marry her boyfriend yet she felt an obligation to please him. She also felt obliged to please his mother who was urging that she continue with the pregnancy and give the child up for adoption. The dynamic operating for the mother was that the younger child in this family was adopted. Part of the boyfriend's urgency to have the child stemmed from his belief that because he was born prematurely in his parent's marriage, that he was conceived out of wedlock, and he too might have been aborted.

The difficulty for the patient herself in terminating the pregnancy probably had to do with the unconscious reason for her becoming pregnant: her need to compensate for her early maternal deprivation. The patient's parents were divorced when she was 3 years old. After a brief period of living with her alcoholic mother, she was given to her father to raise. The patient reasoned that if she gave the baby to her boyfriend she would be repeating an act which she resented. Her unconscious motivation in having the child was to give it the love and responsible mothering that she desperately wanted for herself. Thus, through identification with the child, she could make up for the emotional deprivation she suffered. It was the realization that she was in no position to do so that convinced her to terminate the pregnancy. The brief period of therapy during this crisis seemed to offer enough emotional supports to enable her to follow through with her decision to have the abortion.

CASE 2

A 37-year-old, married woman with two sons ages 6 and 8 had been in treatment for 1 year when she became pregnant. Shortly before marrying her husband, she had an illegal abortion. At that time, neither partner wanted a child. She did not recall any depression or guilt following the abortion, just a feeling of great relief in being able to obtain a medically safe one.

The couple had not planned on having a third child. The pregnancy occurred at a time when they were having marital problems. Although various fantasies about having a girl were elicited, both felt it would be an error to have another child. In addition to the marital difficulties, and some financial pressure, the patient was just beginning to reestablish herself professionally—an important move for her self-esteem. Although the decision to abort seemed wise, the patient became very depressed after the abortion. The following dreams illustrate the depth of her depression and guilt.

Two days after the abortion:

> I was looking for a very young child. I asked everyone if they saw the child. The search went on forever. After years someone said that he knew where the child was. In a large house. I tore

through it, looking. I found *her* in the upper floor. She wasn't a child anymore. She was a grown adult. I remember not saying anything. She turned to me and said, "I could have been a great artist, but you didn't let me be." I tore out of the house without her. She stayed. I was hysterical.

One week after the abortion:

I was watching a group of people leave a funeral chapel. Some of the women were carrying flashlights . . . used to revive those who felt faint. Next I remember standing on the shore watching them put the casket on a raft with a small, delicate, bouquet of flowers on top and it drifted slowly out to sea.

I was told by someone of Mary Reid's funeral which was to be the next day. I remember being very surprised that she had died, and couldn't imagine how the funeral could be so soon since I had just seen her that afternoon and she was perfectly fine. The person who told me about the funeral informed me that it was a suicide, and a surprise to everyone.

Two months after the abortion:

I was passing shops with an urgency to get somewhere. I walked down steps into a grocery. I came to a shelf of small jars of baby food. I put loads in the basket. Someone said you can't have those. I left them and had a feeling of panic and ran out of the store.

Four months after the abortion:

I was in a hospital. I was given a tube to put in my vagina and suction something out. I was left alone and suctioned out a lot of blood in a jar.

One year after the abortion:

I dreamt of being pregnant. I was feeling great and going into the hospital to deliver and to see the baby born. It was natural

childbirth and it was a red-haired girl. I remember desperately
wanting to take it home with me, and being told that I couldn't.
I had the feeling of overwhelming sadness and woke up crying.

This case illustrates several points. I have observed that
women who abort after having children seem to suffer greater
discomfort than women who have not borne children. This
patient "knew" the "potential" she was aborting. She now had
two very talented children so she could concretize the "third
child" in the other children's image.

The *loss* from an abortion might be rearoused years after
the event. For example, another woman began to suffer enormous regret and guilt some 20 years after she had an abortion.
She had two grown children and one younger child. The discussion of abortion reform in the newspapers activated memories
and feelings about her own abortion. Although she partially
compensated for the loss by having the third child, when she
was close to 40 years old, she regreted the abortion. She had no
conscious feeling of loss or guilt at the time of the abortion.
When she came to treatment she was haunted by the idea of the
"lost child." Here again, the patient's feelings of loss were not
felt until she had something to compare the loss to.

The sense of loss after an abortion, where it is present,
frequently is related to whatever hopes and fantasies the pregnancy represents. In case 2, the possibility of having a third
child and the fantasy of a daughter were lost. In other cases,
the abortion could symbolize the loss of a lover, the loss of the
hope of a marriage and motherhood, the loss of a fantasy of
one's importance to a lover, the loss of a relationship, and so
forth. The following case illustrates more of these points.

CASE 3

A 38-year-old, divorced woman, with two teenage children
became pregnant while in intensive treatment. Her current love

relationship was in crisis and she hoped the pregnancy would bring her lover closer to her. Although she was careless about the use of contraceptives, she did not consciously plan to become pregnant. The lover experienced the pregnancy as another of this woman's demands and pleas to be taken care of. Rather than come closer, he withdrew during this period which led to the dissolution of the relationship. She viewed the rejection as one more instance of his lack of ability to commit himself to her. She was able to withdraw from the relationship after the abortion with some depression related to the loss of the relationship, yet with considerable relief. The abortion crisis helped the patient finally resolve what to do about the relationship.

CASE 4

A 32-year-old woman had the following dream 11 years after a self-induced abortion.

> I was in my old home town with two girlfriends and about to go horseback riding. We got to the place after walking a long time. I went into the place with the horses. I felt some anxiety. We couldn't get a horse. Then some lady came over and handed me a bundle wrapped in a sheet and blankets, like a baby, although I couldn't see the baby. I was delighted to hold it. Then the distressing part. When I opened the bundle, just to take a look, there was a kid there and it looked like it was shrinking. Like it was wasting away and I wanted the mother to come and take it away before it would die in my arms. I didn't want to be responsible for it. The more I looked, the more anxious I got.

Following the abortion, the patient's mother buried the 5-month fetus in a shoe box. In associations to the dream, she commented that the baby in the dream looked like the fetus she aborted. The abortion was disturbing because, as she put it, "it was like delivering an unborn child." She had an enormous sense of unfinished business about the pregnancy and abortion and still periodically made contact with the man she became pregnant by, hoping in some way to "undo" that event. When she had intercourse with him, she did not use contraceptives. If she became pregnant, she planned to keep the child and raise it. At times, her guilt became overwhelming, and the sense of loss increased with the passing years. When seen in treatment she was 35-years-old, getting a divorce, and anxious lest she never have children. In the interim years, her mother died and her favorite brother was killed in a motorcycle accident. Having a child would, she felt to some extent, make up for these various other losses.

CASE 5

A 34-year-old graduate student, living with a man she intended to marry, became pregnant by another man when she was feeling distant from her boyfriend. Her only conscious anxiety about the abortion was related to the anesthetic. She had heard that the local anesthetic was painful and so she arranged to have a general anesthetic. After the abortion, she felt relief. She had not spoken of it for 2 years when then she felt some sense of loss and guilt. At that time, she announced that she would eventually be punished for the abortion because she "interrupted the natural sex progression of children." Therefore, she would not give birth to a male, the sex she preferred, but rather to the less desired female child.

This patient tended to dissociate from her feelings about the abortion. Although she spoke of just wanting to get the abortion over with and subsequently of the great relief she felt after the abortion, her behavior and dreams during this period indicated other more powerful reactions. She expressed considerable anger at my being away on vacation when she had the abortion, at a girlfriend for being in Europe at that time, and at the man who impregnated her for not paying for the abortion and for rejecting her. Also she focused on being told not to eat

it was evaluated that the pregnant woman might commit suicide were she to continue with the pregnancy. With the old laws, the psychiatrist was often in a position of a struggle with his or her conscience, personal values, and professional ethics. Although the new laws free the psychiatrist of the decision-making role, he or she and other mental health workers still have a crucial role in helping the pregnant woman to understand her abortion decision and integrate the decision and its psychological consequences into her sense of self. The cases presented illustrate that profound emotional experiences are sometimes associated with becoming pregnant and terminating the pregnancy. The variety of feelings accompanying an abortion points to the fact that, as in many human experiences, complex and opposing emotions can be experienced simultaneously. Awareness of the complex psychological reactions involved in becoming pregnant and choosing abortion can help the woman and society to better cope with and to make more meaningful adjustments and decisions regarding the experience.

chapter 3

PSYCHOLOGICAL ASPECTS OF CONTRACEPTIVE USE IN TEENAGE GIRLS

Julie Spain

> It cannot be denied that contraceptive measures become a necessity in married life at some time or other, and theoretically it would be one of the greatest triumphs of mankind, one of the most tangible liberations from the bondage of nature to which we are subject, were it possible to raise the responsible act of procreation to the level of a voluntary and intentional act, and to free it from its entanglement with an indispensable satisfaction of a natural desire. (Freud, 1898, p. 238)

One of the distinguishing features of modern life is the increased ability to separate sex from procreation. In traditional societies, conception is largely an uncontrolled, fateful concomitant of the expression of sexual desires. Questions of whether or not to have children, how many to have, and when to have them are uncommon. In our society, on the other hand, widespread knowledge of contraception enables us to raise such

I would like to thank the Teen Clinic Staff, Hoboken Family Planning Program, Inc., Hoboken, New Jersey and Herbert Nechin, Ph.D., City University of New York for their assistance in this research.

issues and to handle them. Many studies (e.g. Hill et al., 1959; Rainwater, 1960; Ryder, 1969; USBC, 1973) show that most men and women have definite ideas about the number of children they want and also about when they want to have them. Similarly, many adolescents, however unclear they may be about the future, do know that they do not want children during their teenage years (Presser, 1974). With them, however, the ability to act on these desires—or, in Freud's words, to act intentionally—seems to be at least partially determined by subjective beliefs about their capacity to control their destinies, rather than by the objective *facts* of this possibility.

The availability of contraception as an option and the changes in adolescent sexual mores requires large adjustments in people's attitudes and beliefs. Adolescents, in particular, are in a transitional stage: changes in sexual mores have not always been followed by psychological shifts that would allow contraception to be viewed as a real option. The gap between increased sexual activity and effective contraceptive use in adolescents has resulted in pregnancies for 10 percent of female teenagers. Approximately 11 million teenagers, more than one-half of the teenage population in the United States, have had sexual intercourse, and 1 million 15-to 19-year-olds and 30,000 girls younger than 15 become pregnant annually (Guttmacher, 1976; Jaffe & Dryfoos, 1976). The fact that most of these pregnancies are unplanned and many are unwanted after they occur shows that adolescents who are sexually active are not using, or are ineffectively using, contraception. Thus, teenage pregnancy reflects not a conscious choice for procreation, but rather the difficulty adolescents face in exerting control over their lives.

The sexually active teenagers' pattern of contraceptive use is subject to a wide range of influences. Knowledge about reproduction and contraception, and accessibility of family planning service are obvious prerequisites to effective use. Many well-informed teenagers, however, some of whom even possess methods of birth control, are unsuccessful in preventing pregnancy. Research in the 1950's investigated whether difficulty in preventing unwanted children was caused primarily by an absence of information about contraception. One study (Hill et al., 1959) found that in an outpatient sample of 3000 Puerto Rican women who were ineffective in using contraception, less than 0.5 percent claimed to be unaware of birth control, while women between the ages of 15 and 19 knew an average of 2.5 methods. More recent studies (Cobliner, 1971; Fujita et al., 1971; Furstenberg, 1971; Kane et al., 1974; Kane & Lachenbruch, 1973) have provided additional evidence that the primary determinant of women's difficulties in preventing unwanted pregnancies is not lack of knowledge about contraception.

Since family planning programs have become increasingly accessible to adolescents, it becomes clearer that many teenagers who actually obtained methods of birth control are nonetheless high risks for pregnancy. Research focusing on the psychological aspects of this phenomenon has provided two different perspectives to explain ineffective contraceptive use. One perspective is based on the psychoanalytic tradition, and explains unplanned pregnancy as a motivated phenomenon. The pregnancy is sometimes viewed as an "acting out" of oedipal conflicts of adolescence. The teenage girl uses the pregnancy and the child as a way of maintaining the fantasy of her special relationship with her father (Cobliner, 1974). In other cases, the pregnancy is described as the girl's attempt to maintain her own infantile dependency on her mother (Babikian & Goldman, 1971; Blos, 1969; Deutsch, 1967; Schaffer & Pine, 1972). Through her identification with her child, the teenage girl is able to "regain" the feeling of early nurturing as her own mother cares for her child. In these cases, the pregnancy is generally viewed as a "regressive" phenomenon. For a smaller group of adolescents, the pregnancy is a "progressive" solution to the conflicts of adolescent. These girls use the experience of childbearing and childrearing to resolve earlier conflicts and to move on to constructively dealing with tasks appropriate to adolescent and adult development.

A composite clinical picture emerges of the girls described by this psychoanalytic perspective. The girl's mother had her own difficulties with childrearing that was frequently reflected in her inability to provide consistent nurturing. The care provided during infancy and childhood was either insufficent, leaving the child with a sense of deprivation, or overindulgent. These girls then enter adolescence with deficits in their sense of time, reality testing, and ability to tolerate frustration. Therefore, normal adolescent conflicts are particularly difficult for them to handle.

The second perspective in the literature describes teenage pregnancy as an unmotivated, accidental consequence of sexual intercourse. The inability to use contraception effectively is seen as stemming from issues other than the wish to become pregnant. One example of research within this tradition (Cobliner, 1974; 1976) explains deficits in adolescent's cognitive development as the barrier to their using contraception effectively. According to this theory, many teenagers have not reached the stage of operative thinking in which they are able to imagine the future. They have no ideas about future consequences by which to judge present behavior. The decision to use contraception, which is predicated on this judgment, is therefore not within their scope. The study reported in this chapter draws on findings from both these perspectives.

CONDITIONS OF THE STUDY

Twenty-one girls, aged 14 to 18, were interviewed for this study. They were randomly selected from a Teen Clinic in a typical family planning program. Information on their contraceptive and sexual history was obtained by a Registered Nurse. Based on this information, they then were assigned to either the ineffective or effective contraceptive user group. Each subgroup included black, white, and Puerto Rican girls, all from the lower socioeconomic classes. The groups differed in their religious compositions. While both groups had girls who described themselves as Catholic or Protestant, Baptists were found only in the ineffective contraceptive group.

The data were obtained from a structured interview that was tape-recorded, from forced choice questions that were read to the girls because of their low reading levels, and from eight cards from the Thematic Apperception Test. There were four areas of investigation, which focused on the future and planning for it, on sexuality and sexual decision making, on locus of control and coping mechanisms, and on peer group procreational patterns. The findings of other research and clinical work with similar girls led to the decision to concentrate on these areas. The quotations cited in the chapter are excerpted from the taped interviews.

FUTURE AND PLANNING

Adolescents' concept of time is related to their use of contraception. Teenage girls with the ability to distinguish between the present and the future, to imagine themselves in the future, and then to logically link their present behavior to realistic future goals tend to be effective contraceptive users. These effective users charateristically have thought about the future and understand that their behavior has consequences. Their descriptions of the present reflect a self-consciousness and emerging sense of self.

Marcia, 17-years-old, began using contraception one month prior to her first sexual experience. Excerpts from the interview with her illustrate that she projects to the future and sees planning as an integral part of her life. In response to the question, "Do you have other thoughts about the future?" she said:

I'd like to be very well off. I'd like to go into hematology research. I'd like to get married and I'm not too sure about kids. If I do it will only be two and I'd like to live in New York City in a large apartment. . . . I hope I'm happy. I think if I continue and become a doctor, I will be happy. . . . Over the summer I worked at Mt. Sinai as a volunteer in a lab where the doctor is a hematologist. I helped the technicians and I really enjoyed myself and what I was doing. I thought I would think about it once I got to college and planned a major.

Question: Have you thought about the things you might do to make this all happen?

First college. I realize it's a lot of years, but I want it. I know it will all happen. I couldn't see myself doing anything else. I'm really interested in it and I'm a rather strong willed person. I think I can make it through the school years.

Marcia's sense of conviction about the future contrasts sharply with that of girls who are ineffective contraception users. These girls often express confusion about the concept of time, have difficulty imagining themselves in the future, and have either no goals or unrealistic ones that bear no relationship to present activities.

Roxanne, a 16-year-old, first had intercourse at age 13, had an abortion at 15, and was not using contraception at the time of the interview, although she was sexually active. In the interview, she expressed how disappointments and losses instilled a sense of hopelessness which became translated into a negative or deterministic view of the future. It was as if her only decision was to make no decisions. She virtually denied the future as being connected organically to her or in any way within her control. Roxanne had dropped out of school, saying that she would not return to school and that she never thought about it. In response to "Do you ever have thoughts about when you'll be 21?" she said "no" and continued:

A lot of times I plan things and they never happen. I knew this guy, we're not going together now. We planned to get an apartment, we planned to get engaged and then we broke off for a month. That's why I don't plan anything. I had my hopes all up. When my niece was in the hospital, I said—"When she comes out that we would do this," and she had pneumonia. She passed away. That's why I don't plan things. If they happen, they happen, you know.

Another girl who was high risk for pregnancy conveyed a childlike way of thinking about the future. In response to "Do you ever have thoughts about the future?", Michelle said:

Dreams! I always wanted to be an acrobat and then I thought about getting married. I was never smart, but dreamt of being an acrobat, an ice skater.

Question: What kinds of dreams do you have now?

Just about Billy, my boyfriend.

Question: Do you think you'll be an acrobat?

No.

Michelle continued by saying that she never thought about the future: "I mainly think about what I'm doing now. It's too hard to think about the future."

Other research (Cochrane et al., 1973; Goldsmith et al., 1972; Kar, 1971; Keller et al., 1970; Miller, 1964) is in agreement with this finding that differences in teenagers' attitudes towards the future and planning are reflected in differences in patterns of contraceptive use.

Feelings about Sex

Feelings about sex, the nature of sexual contact, and motivation for sex are all related to the teenagers' patterns of contraceptive use. Most teenagers have hesitation about their initial sexual contact, experiencing some guilt and conflict about these experiences. The manner in which the teenager handles the guilt and conflict has an impact on whether or not she utilizes contraception. Girls who are aware of their guilt and discomfort and do not try to deny it tend to be effective in their use of contraception. The effective contraceptive users generally have sex when they want it and enjoy both the physical and emotional aspects of their sexual contact. They feel relatively comfortable with their sexuality, expressing little embarassment about the choices they have made to have intercourse.

Joan, a 17-year-old who used contraception prior to her first sexual experience at age 15, frankly described her initial hesitation, but also revealed a basic sense of self respect which resulted in her sense of choice about her experiences.

> Before I was 15 I don't think I could have handled it. I just know I wasn't ready—I guess mentally. I guess I thought sex was dirty and I guess I didn't care enough about him. But when I did have sex the first time, I knew—it was Christmas Day and I knew it was going to happen. I guess a woman's intuition. I was so happy I cried. I never felt closer to anybody in my life. I have sex now because of the pleasure too, but I'm not much with words and the guy I'm going with now is very quiet and he can't say what's on his mind. It's just our form of expression. I feel so much for him, it's hard to explain, but I love being with him, I love being near him, his ideas I like, the things we've shared—I can't use words.

In contrast, when a sexually active teenager is highly ambivalent or guilty about sex and continues her sexual contact despite these feelings, she is likely to be an ineffective contraceptive user. Dislike of sex and anger at the sexual partner often contribute to teens' resistance to using contraception. The ineffective users express carelessness and thoughtlessness concerning the sexual decision-making process. The needs that are fulfilled through their sexual contact have little or nothing to do with any pleasure in the sexual act itself. For example, a 17-year-old girl said "It makes me feel good because then I'll know that he won't go out and mess around with someone else.

When we have sex that makes me feel good because he came to me and asked me. That's the main feeling, that he came to me." Following intercourse, her boyfriend asked, "How did you like it?" she said "How did I like what?" Denial of the sexual experience itself is typical of girls who do not use contraception.

Jeanette, a 15-year-old with a history of two abortions and sporadic contraceptive use, described the self-denial involved in her decision to have sex.

> I don't know why I had sex the first time, because that's when I was a virgin. He kept telling me how we were going to get married and stuff like that and how I shouldn't be afraid. He thought I was another type of girl who goes around with a lot of guys and I told him I was a virgin. He told me I was a liar. I said "If you don't want to believe me then don't." He said "Are you sure" and I said "Yes." In my mind I said what am I going to be shy for because I knew him for four years. So what I did was say "I'll prove it to you." So we had sex and then he said "Now I believe you . . ." They start trying to kiss your mouth first, that's when the girls start getting hot. You feel like pushing them away. They want to feel enjoyment but they don't care how you feel. Me, I don't know what they're doing. If I tell him, you know how guys are, they start getting mad. I don't really like sex that much. You get sick or you can get any kind of things.

Angela, another ineffective contraceptive user, in sharing feelings similar to Jeanette, demonstrates the extent of this pattern.

> I had this boyfriend, he started talking and I said, no, no, no, because I was 13, and then when I became 14 I started liking him more and more, but I couldn't get myself to do it. I would sit and think and then when I turned 15 he said "If you like me the way you say you like me then you'll do it." In my mind I said, no, no, no. Then one day, I just let it happen. In my mind I was saying no, my mother, my mother. I don't get nothing out of it. I don't want it but the men want it. I don't know what they get out of it because all I get out of it is a mess. I say no, but then

sometimes you can't say no. It's a mess. I was stupid to do it in the first place. I just let it happen. Sometimes I just look and say no and then I say no so many times that he will get mad at me. It was all so messy.

Other studies (Fujita, 1971; Goldsmith et al., 1972; Kane & Lachenbruch, 1973; Lieberman, 1964) confirm that contraception can easily become the target for the expression of negative feelings about sex. In addition, guilt about sex can lead teenagers to unconsciously rationalize their sexual activity as a means to an end; the end being reproduction. By not using contraception, they are giving their sexual activity a built-in justification.

ATTITUDES ABOUT CONTROL AND COPING MECHANISMS

The effectiveness of contraceptive use is also determined by whether the teenager believes that her life is shaped by internal controls, such as her own behavior, or by external ones, such as God and fate. The girls who are successful in using contraception can identify the alternatives that are available and can act in response to them. They believe themselves to be in control of their own lives, while demonstrating the understanding and emotional stability necessary for such a belief. When directly questioned they describe themselves as the most important influence in what happens to them, and they are confident about their ability to make things work. They think through problem situations, look for solutions, and consciously try to prevent recurrences.

In describing her educational plans, Catherine, a 16-year-old effective contraceptive user, reveals these characteristics.

I'm in the eleventh grade now and I graduate next year. School is okay. I can dig school when I want to. I have to discipline myself sometimes. School itself, the system is okay. You can't wear dungarees or sneakers and I like that. I can deal with it, even though I was stubborn when I got there. They tamed me alot so I can follow the rules. I have no trouble at all getting along. There's time for play and time for work. You have to say I have to get this done and this done and then I play. Last year there were times when I goofed off alot and when I saw my report card I said "Well let me stop because I want to go to college."

I really do. I played first and second semester, but third I got down to business. I really want to go to college but the money situation is difficult. Years ago I was saying "What the hell, what's the use of college?" Now I see a difference. Even it I have to take out loans I'm going. By the time I'm 26 I should have the career part the way I want it. After about four years of marriage I'll start having kids.

It is not as if Catherine does not have problems, but she clearly identifies them and explores alternative ways of dealing with them by reflecting on her past. In contrast, the teenagers who are ineffective contraceptive users identify external sources as controlling them and therefore do not seek alternatives or reflect on ways of coping more productively. They are unskilled at talking about how they feel, what they want or how they can cope with difficult situations. Their ability to think things through before acting is limited.

Evelyn, an 18-year-old ineffective user, for example, identifies her problems in school and the solutions as outside of herself.

No, I'm not in school now. I dropped out in my third year. I liked school alot. I had too many problems when I quit school —fights with other girls, the girls used to pick on me. My mother used to have to go to court for me, for my playing hooky. I came out all right, my mother used to talk to me: "try to be good until you're 16, when you're 16 I'll take you out of school." I started night school. I can't really say whether I'll finish, because I don't really know, if I do or if I don't. I can't really do anything about it. I thought in a way so many of the problems I've been seeing that I hope I don't go through them. Like if I have a problem I just go to my mother. She says "do this . . . do that. . . ."

> Like some people get into your problems—don't be this, don't
> be that. Some people give you good advice and some don't give
> you no good advice. They mess you up and mess up your life.

Other studies (Hill et al., 1959; Keller et al., 1970; Lundy, 1972; MacDonald, 1970; Meyerowitz & Malev, 1973) have similarly found that passive and fatalistic attitudes, difficulty with planning, and an external locus of control are all associated with high risk for pregnancy among teenagers.

PEER GROUP AND MOTIVES FOR PROCREATION

The patterns of childbearing within the teen's peer group and the nature of her involvement with her peer group bear some relationship to success in using contraception. In this study, the differences between the effective and ineffective users did not reach statistical significance on all measures of motives for procreation. The following discussion is based on trends and clinical example.

Both the effective and ineffective users know other girls their age who have been pregnant and have had children. The effective users generally do not reveal wishes for children, however, often taking a harsh and critical view of their peers who are mothers. These girls' sense of individuality or autonomy seems to enable them to differentiate themselves from peer group norms that favor procreation.

Allison, an 18-year-old effective contraceptive user is clear that she does not want children until accomplishing her educational goals. She said of her peers:

> When I see someone who is my own age and pregnant I feel sorry
> for them. Plus I think about how they haven't begun to live
> themselves, and they have another life that they have to worry
> about. When I see someone who looks fairly complete as a
> person and they're happy about it and their face looks happy,
> then I'm happy for them. . . . I saw Sara on the avenue with her

baby and I had this feeling that she was treating it like a doll. It was just like—look at the baby and I don't really think she thought about it. . . . I think it's a sin. To bring a baby into the world and not be sure of yourself, you're just stretching out too much and creating too much responsibility.

Kim, a 16-year-old effective contraceptive user, describes wishes that she does have for a child. While drawn towards pregnancy, however, she is not overwhelmed by jealousy of peers. Rather than denying her wishes she carefully examines her impulse to have a child and is then able to open herself to the experiences of others from whom she can learn.

They become pregnant because they see everyone else pregnant. They say things like, "Oh I wish I had a baby." They think it's easy to have a baby. They say, "No I can support it." I don't want no welfare supporting my kid. I want to support my kid myself. I see a lot of young kids pregnant. They see older women pregnant and they think it's easy to have a kid. I say yeah, it's nice to have a kid if you have money. If you don't have money why have a kid. I was going to get pregnant. Then I said "No, I have no money, I have no home. When my kid grows up I don't want my kid to be living in my mother's home.

In contrast, the ineffective users appear to be particularly embedded in a peer culture where pregnancy is the norm. Babies and pregnancy are seen as a fated accidental part of life. At the same time, they become a way by which girls can fill an emptiness or possess something. Laura, a 17-year-old ineffective user said:

Oh, I want me one. Everytime I see someone pregnant I'll be touching their stomach. I'll say, "Oh, I want me one so bad." That's what makes me think I want me one. If I don't see no one with a stomach then it don't bother me.

Laura does not have particularly more contact with a peer culture where pregnancy is the norm than do the two other girls. Rather, her sense of autonomy is not established, so her wishes are reflective of her immediate culture. Evelyn, an 18-year-old ineffective contraceptive user is clearly ambivalent about the place of a child in her life.

> I get a lot of feelings when I see my friend's pregnant. In a way I start thinking of myself, she's so young, why does she do that; she won't be able to party, will be stuck in the house. When I see a girl like that I think about how I'll be having the same problems too. I won't be able to party. . . . I see them pregnant and I say to myself they're younger than me, man. I would like to have a kid and they already have one. Why couldn't I have one if they could have one already. So could I. I see them and I say to myself in a way they mistreat the babies and when they hit them when they're so small, and I say to myself God gives kids to the bad people and to the good people, the people who want them, don't have them. When I have a kid I'll be so happy. I really want one.

Further research is necessary to explore the trends discussed here about the influence of procreational motives on contraceptive use. These findings suggest that there may be subgroups of girls. One group of ineffective users may, in fact, have unconscious wishes for procreation and therefore are resistant to contraception. Another group may have no interest in childbearing during their teenage years, and may have difficulty with contraception for the reasons stated in the three previous sections.

CONCLUSION

In general, the girls who are ineffective contraceptive users seem to feel that they have very little in life, nothing to look forward to, and no sense or hope of a tomorrow. They take a stance of passively responding to and fulfilling the demands, pressures, and sometimes the pleasures of others in their day-today-functioning. Pregnancy to them is not life or fulfillment but represents the possibility of having something. The baby often seems like a *thing*. In contrast, the effective contraceptive users show an interest and excitement about experiencing the richness of growing up with a relative openness to difficulties and conflicts. They seem to have a sense of control over their lives that enables them to speculate about their roles in the present and their potential in the future. Childbearing is seen as another challenge, as something special which they view their peers as abusing. In fact, they respond to pregnancy and childbearing as they do to their sexual activity, as a process in which their own feelings and needs are important.

Modern contraceptive methods contain the potential for freeing men and women from unwanted pregnancy and children. In the most general terms, however, this research has shown that the use of contraception is very much entangled with not only sexual feelings and behavior but many other aspects of living. The availability of effective methods of contraception is an essential part of the process of controlling and planning procreation, but responding to this availability involves a complex interaction of personal, interpersonal, and other factors which are not within the scope of chemical or mechanical interventions. Professionals can be most effective when they respond to the whole person in their assessment of adolescents as risks for pregnancy and in the subsequent counseling process.

REFERENCES

Babikian, H., & Goldman, A. A study in teenage pregnancy. *American Journal of Psychiatry,* 1971, *128,* 755–760.

Blos, P. Three typical constellations in female delinquency. In O. Pollak & A. S. Friedman (Eds.), *Family dynamics and female sexual delinquency.* Palo Alto: Science and Behavior Books, 1969.

Cobliner, W. G. Pregnancy in the single adolescent girl; The role of cognitive functions. *Journal of Youth and Adolescence,* 1974, *3,* 17–29.

Cobliner, W. G. Teenage out-of wedlock pregnancy: A phenomenon of many dimensions. *Bulletin of New York Academy of Medicine,* 1976, *46,* 438–447.

Cochrane, C. M., Vincent, C. E., Haney, C. A. & Michielute, R. Motivational determinants of family planning clinic attendance. *Journal of Psychology,* 1973, *84,* 33–43.

Deutsch, H. *Selected problems of adolescence.* New York: International Universities Press, 1967.

Freud, S. (1898) Sexuality in the aetiology of the neuroses. In *Sigmund Freud Collected papers. Volume I.* New York: Basic Books, 1959.

Furstenberg, F. E. Birth Control experience among pregnant adolescents: The process of unplanned parenthood. *Social Problems,* 1971, *19,* 192–203.

Guttmacher Institute. *11 million teenagers—What can be done about the epidemic of adolescent pregnancies in the United States?* New York: Planned Parenthood Federation of America, Inc., 1976.

Fujita, B. N., Wagner, N. N., & Pion, R. J. Contraceptive use among single college students. *American Journal of Obstetrics and Gynecology,* 1971, 109, 184–193.

Goldsmith, S., Gabrielson, M. O., Gabrielson, I., Mathews, V. & Potts, L. Teenagers, sex and contraception. *Family Planning Perspectives,* 1972, *4,* 32–38.

Hill, R., Stycos, J. M., & Back, K. W. *The Family and population control.* New Haven: College and University Press, 1959.

Jaffe, F. S., & Dryfoos, J. G. Fertility control services for adolescents: Access and utilization. *Family Planning Perspectives,* 1976, *8,* 167–175.

Kane, F. J., and Lachenbruch, P. A. Adolescent pregnancy: A study of aborters and nonaborters. *American Journal of Orthopsychiatry,* 1973, *43,* 796–803.

Kane, F. J., Moan, C. A., & Bolling, B. Motivational factors in pregnant adolescents. *Disease of Nervous System,* 1974, *35,* 131–134.

Kar, S. B. Individual aspirations as related to early and late acceptance of contraception. *Journal of Social Psychology,* 1971, *83,* 235–245.

Keller, A. B., Sims, J. H., Henry, W. E., & Crawford, T. J. Psychological sources of "resistance" to family planning. *Merrill-Palmer Quarterly,* 1970, *16,* 286–302.

Lieberman, J. E. Preventive psychiatry and family planning. *Journal of Marriage and the Family,* 1964, *26,* 471–477.

Lundy, J. R. Some personality correlates of contraceptive use among unmarried female college students. *The Journal of Psychology,* 1972, *80,* 9–14.

MacDonald, A. P., Jr. Internal-external locus of control and the practice of birth control, *Psychological Reports,* 1970, *27,* 206.

Miller, W. *Personality factors in premarital pregnancy: Data analysis.* (Final Report) National Institute of Child Health and Human Development,

Department of Health, Education and Welfare (Contract #NO 1-HD-52804), 1964.

Meyerowitz, J. H., & Malev, J. S. Pubescent attitudinal correlates antecedent to adolescent illegitimate pregnancy. *Journal of Youth and Adolescence,* 1973, *2,* 251–258.

Presser, H. B. Early motherhood: Ignorance or bliss? *Family Planning Perspectives,* 1974, *6,* 8–14.

Rainwater, L. *And the poor get children.* Chicago: Quadrangle, 1960.

Ryder, N. B., & Westoff, C. F. Relationship among intended, expected, desired and ideal family size: United States 1965. Independent Study for the Center for Population Research, 1969.

Schaffer, C., & Pine, F. Pregnancy, abortion and the developmental tasks of adolescence. *Journal of the American Academy of Child Psychiatry,* 1972, *11,* 511–536.

United States Bureau of the Census. Birth expectations of American wives: June 1973. *Current Population Reports,* Series P-20, No. 24.

Young, L. *Out of wedlock.* New York: McGraw-Hill, 1954.

chapter 4

UNDERSTANDING ADOLESCENT PREGNANCY

Andrea Marks

Adolescent pregnancy is a subject of paramount national interest and concern. Discussions of its precursors and consequences are featured repeatedly in newspapers, magazines, television spots, as well as community and political arenas. The hard facts are that approximately 1 million adolescent girls become pregnant each year, or 1 out of every 10 13- to 19-year-old females. The birth rate among all adolescents has decreased since the mid-1960s, but to a lesser degree than it has for older women, and the number of births to adolescents in the 13- to 17-year-old cohort actually has increased slightly. In 1976, 600,000 adolescent pregnancies resulted in live births, a rate surpassed by very few western industrialized nations (Monthly Vital Statistics Report, 1977; 1978).

The number of births to adolescents might be even higher were it not for the liberalization of abortion and the increased availability of contraceptives to teenagers which have occurred within this decade. About 300,000 adolescents obtain abortions annually, representing one-third of the total abortions performed (Center for Disease Control, 1977). It has been estimated that an additional 680,000 adolescent pregnancies are prevented each year through effective use of contraceptives (Zelnick & Kantner, 1978).

Ninety percent of adolescents who bear infants keep and care for their babies, often in the home of their own mother. The impact of such an event on the adolescent's own dynamic state of psychosocial development can only be dramatic.

Understanding adolescent pregnancy is an important goal for all who work with teenagers. This includes understanding the normal psychosocial developmental issues of adolescents, their styles of contraception utilization and decision making regarding abortion, and the unique psychological impact of a pregnancy and early parenthood on such a young person. With these tools, we may attempt to help our patients or clients to prevent unwanted pregnancies, to make personally well-suited choices at the point of discovering an early pregnancy, and to deal effectively with the stressful events of an abortion or of pregnancy and parenthood.

PSYCHOSOCIAL DEVELOPMENT

The psychosocial process of adolescence has no precise onset and no certain sign of completion. It generally begins around the time of initial pubescent physical changes and continues until a reasonable sense of self is achieved. Adolescence as a developmental stage has gripped the curiosity of numerous authors who have described it from psychoanalytic (Blos, 1962), social (Erikson, 1963), and anthropological (Mead, 1928) viewpoints.

There are at least three basic tasks of adolescence which in concert contribute to a stable adult identity: establishing independence from parents and family, feeling at ease with one's gender role and sexuality, and formulating a plan toward becoming a contributing member of society. The adolescent approaches these tasks at home with the family, in the peer group, and at school or work. The degree of mastering each task and the nature of the struggle change as the teenager passes through early, middle, and late stages of adolescence.

The early adolescent experiences rapid growth and pubescent changes. His or her body not only begins to look different but also acts in new ways, as the onset of menstruation or ejaculation signal reproductive potential. New sexual sensations emerge, but the early adolescent characteristically remains most intensely involved in activities with the same sex peers, when not engrossed totally with self during typical periods of isolation. The struggle for independence begins in faltering earnest during early adolescence. Authority still resides with parents in the young teenager's eyes, but challenging that authority proceeds nonetheless, interspersed with eager cries for nurturing.

The middle adolescent is blessed with enhanced intellectual potential. The newly found capacity for abstract thinking facilitates close friendships for the sharing of feelings and ideas. Physical growth is much less rapid and the adolescent's increasing comfort with his or her body allows for the onset of sexual experimentation with the opposite sex. For the middle adolescent, authority resides with the peer group, which may provide a sense of security in the face of newly shed family supports, but may also become a source of pressure into involvement with drugs, tobacco, alcohol, or unprotected sexual activity.

Late adolescence is a time of future planning, when authority resides mostly within the self, and identity is emerging into fuller independence. Rebellion against parents is mellowed by gradual acceptance of them and friendships are selected, not possessed. Heterosexual relationships reflect the needs and commonalities of the involved individuals and are of increased depth and commitment.

Adolescent Sexuality and Contraception

Sexual activity, which includes intercourse, may begin in early, middle, or late adolescence, or beyond the teenage years. The increased prevalence of premarital sexual intercourse, which occurred in the late 1960s and continues into the 1970s, includes adolescents. A 1976 nationwide study (Zelnick & Kantner, 1977) indicated that 55 percent of 19-year-old and 18 percent of 15-year-old females had experienced sexual intercourse. The mean age at first intercourse was 16.2 years, slightly younger than the 16.5 mean found by the same researchers in 1971. The overall rate of sexual intercourse experienced by 15- to 19-year-old females in these same studies was 35 percent in 1976 versus 27 percent in 1971, a prevalence increase of 30 percent. There are data (Hein, 1978) to show that certain populations of adolescent females have a much higher prevalence of sexual experience and younger age at first intercourse.

Much remains to be learned about the sexual behavior of adolescent females, yet our experience has revealed certain patterns that seem to relate to stage of psychosocial development. The sexually active (i.e., experienced with sexual intercourse) early adolescent often is embroiled in severe intrafamilial clashes, school failure, and other forms of acting out or rebellious behavior, which may even be covering up a severe depression. She is more likely to be ignorant of reproductive physiology and anatomy (including her own), and seems to be less likely to experience true sexual pleasure or understanding with a series of partners, with whom she has shallow relationships. Her use of contraceptives is generally quite poor or nonexistent.

Sexual activity during middle adolescence seems less likely to be related to major difficulties at home, and more likely linked to peer pressure or group norms. Knowledge and pleasure are at a higher level, relationships with partners are often monogamous and associated with strong positive feelings, and use of contraceptives is far better by these adolescents whose rapid pubertal changes occurred several years past.

The late adolescent's sexual activity is more a personal decision linked to deeper levels of responsibility and mutuality. Decisions regarding sexual activity, contraception, abortion, and pregnancy tend to relate to a future-oriented life plan.

Few sexually active adolescents (7 percent, state they are seeking to become pregnant (Shah, 1975), and these girls naturally do not practice any form of contraception. A second group is determined not to become pregnant and regularly uses effective birth control. A third cluster does not wish to become pregnant but does not regularly use birth control, and a fourth group states they are not sure or "wouldn't mind" getting pregnant; these adolescents generally do not use contraceptives regularly, if at all. It is the last two groups which especially challenge our understanding. The girls in the third group become pregnant frequently and generally choose abortion. The ambivalent girls in the fourth group are more likely to continue with a pregnancy. The most frequently given reason by 15- to 19-year-old females for not using contraception is that they do not think they could become pregnant, either because it is the wrong time of the month to conceive or their bodies are too young and intercourse too infrequent (Shah, 1975). Yet only 40 percent of this sample knew when ovulation occurred. Fewer girls attributed nonuse of contraception to its unavailability.

Contraceptives available today present a potpourri of problems even to adult women who have been sexually active for years and are comfortable with their matured bodies. For the adolescent, whose "new body" and emerging sexuality are yet to be fully integrated into his or her identity, most contraceptive methods pose even greater difficulties. The condom, foam, and diaphragm must be at hand when needed, which involves planning ahead, contemplating intercourse hours before it occurs, and carrying devices. Actually using these particular methods at the time of intercourse requires touching one's own genitals, which is unappealing to many female adolescents, and communicating adequately with a sexual partner at a time of heightened arousal. The pill and intrauterine device require a long-term commitment to sexual activity and admitting to oneself on a daily or ongoing basis that contraception is a part of life. Such sexual awareness is threatening to many adolescents.

Despite these obstacles, Zelnick and Kantner (1977, 1978) have reported a sharp increase in contraceptive use by adolescent females, and a shift away from the condom, douche, and withdrawal to widespread acceptance of the pill and IUD. We have been impressed by a significant interest in the diaphragm by approximately one-third of our adolescent patients, and long-term effective use of this method by many of them.

Approximately 50 percent of adolescent females are reported to use some form of contraception at the time of first intercourse (Sorenson, 1972; Zelnick & Kantner, 1978). Older adolescents are more likely to do so, and those who start out as contraceptors are more likely to continue with birth control in a consistent manner.

PREGNANCY AND PARENTHOOD

As noted earlier, approximately one million adolescents become pregnant each year. Zelnick and Kantner's (1978) study group of sexually active 15- to 19-year-old females consisted of 27 percent always-, 42 percent sometimes-, and 31 percent never-users of contraceptives. Pregnancy was experienced by 11 percent, 24 percent, and 58 percent of each group, respectively. Among the never-users, 70 percent did not intend to become pregnant. Those teenagers who chose abortion were twice as likely to have used contraception at the time pregnancy occurred than those who chose to continue with the pregnancy.

A newly-discovered pregnancy may be met by shock, dismay, happiness, confusion, fear, guilt, denial, or generally a combination of emotions. Eventually, however, the adolescent must decide whether she wishes to continue with the pregnancy or have an abortion. Sometimes the pregnancy is denied or a decision avoided for so long that abortion no longer remains an option.

For some adolescents the decision is immediately clear; either motherhood or abortion is completely untenable or unwanted and plans can proceed accordingly. For others, an agonizing decision-making process begins, and these teenagers require counseling and support from family members and nonjudgmental health professionals until a reasonable personal decision is reached. We must try to be in touch with the stated and the underlying reasons for a particular leaning or ultimate choice.

Stated reasons for continuing with an unplanned pregnancy include: "I want to have a baby." "I don't believe in abortion." "My boyfriend (or mother) want the baby and will help me," or "I've already had one abortion and am afraid to have another." Reasons generally not stated by the adolescent include loneliness and a search for nurturance through nurturing, a desire to get closer to her own mother or to escape from an intolerable home situation, boredom and failure in school and a wish to find something new to occupy herself, and a need to prove her femaleness. Our impression is that adolescents who choose to continue with a pregnancy, especially the younger adolescents, are more likely to come from crisis-laden families, do poorly in school, and have confused identities with depression and low self-esteem.

Pregnancy at any age is somewhat of a crisis, even when it is fully wished for in a richly supportive setting. For the teenager, pregnancy enters upon the ongoing dynamic and stressful process of adolescent psychosocial development itself. The pregnancy is usually a first one, and often unplanned. Simultaneously, the pregnancy signals the onset of a new life role, either wife-mother or out-of-wedlock mother.

The social consequences of adolescent pregnancy are well-known and include failure to continue education, dependency on welfare, and never marrying. The unique psychological consequences, which are immediate, relate directly to the major developmental issues of adolescence. These include an altered dependency relationship with parents (usually mother), intrusion into early sexual experimentation and age-appropriate peer group relationships and activities, and loss of the primary societal role of student. These jolts can cause anxiety, depression, and feelings of isolation for the very young mother-to-be.

Each family reacts in its own way to the news of an adolescent daughter's pregnancy. Generally an initial period of anger, grief, or confusion is replaced by support, but this very process may retard the degree of emancipation which the teenager has struggled to achieve. The girl who remains at home during a pregnancy and thereafter, experiences increased dependency on her parents for financial aid, living space, and help preparing and caring for an infant. Roles may become blurred, as grandmother acts as the primary caretaker for the infant, sharply diminishing the teenager's self-esteem and ability to grow into a mothering relationship with her own offspring.

The physiologic changes that accompany pregnancy may, for a young girl who has only recently experienced rapid pubertal changes, place an extra degree of stress on her sense of body integrity. New physical limitations of pregnancy, as well as social restrictions placed by parents, schools, friends, or the adolescent herself tend to isolate her from her peer group. The putative father may or may not be part of her life anymore, and if he is not, the normal fears of impending labor, delivery, and motherhood cannot be allayed by the presence of a loving father-to-be. Rather abruptly, the adolescent is no longer a student who plays or pursues her own interests during evenings and weekends, and is free to experiment with different people and new games and to plan for a future with options. Many pregnant teenagers seem to have little interest in such pursuits, mainly because they have been unsuccessful with them in the past. Pregnancy and motherhood are expected by them to provide a new sense of achievement and fulfillment.

Can any good result from an adolescent pregnancy? Can a teenager mature as a result of this experience and find herself better off? Can families benefit and infants do well? Can failure cycles be interrupted? The answers to these important questions are not fully known, but certainly those of us who work with teenage mothers know that some of them do well. Adolescent prenatal programs and follow-up programs for young mothers and their babies are trying to address the unique problems which pregnancy and motherhood create for adolescents (McAnarney, 1978; Perkins, 1978). The goal of these efforts has been to impact on the negative social and psychologial sequelae that have already been discussed. The success of these programs has been slow and uncertain, but for now, working with pregnant and mothering adolescents proceeds enthusiastically.

REFERENCES

Blos, P. *On adolescence: A psychoanalytic interpretation.* New York: The Free Press, 1962.

Center for Disease Control. *Abortion surveillance: annual summary, 1975.* Atlanta, 1977.

Erikson, E. H. *Childhood and society.* New York: Norton, 1963.

Hein, K., Cohen, M. I., Marks, A., Schonberg, S. K., Meyer, M., & McBride A. Age at first intercourse among homeless adolescent females. *Journal of Pediatrics,* 1978, *93,* 147–148.

McAnarney, E. R., Roghmann, K. J., Adam, B. N., Tatelbaum, R. C., Kash, C., Coulter, M., Plume, M., & Charney, E. Obstetric, neonatal and psychosocial outcome of pregnant adolescents. *Pediatrics,* 1978, *61,* 199–205.

Mead, M. *Coming of age in Samoa.* New York: Dell, 1928.

Monthly Vital Statistics Report, Natality statistics from the National Center for Health Statistics: Teenage Childbearing: United States, 1966–1975 (DHEW Publication No. (HRA) 77-1120, Vol 26, No. 5 Suppl). Washington, D.C., U.S. Government Printing Office, 1977.

Monthly Vital Statistics Report: Advance Report: Final natality statistics, 1976 (DHEW Pub. No. (PHS) 78-1120. Vol. 26, No. 12, Suppl). Washington, D.C., U.S. Government Printing Office, 1978.

Perkins, R. P., Nakashima, I. I., Mullin, M., Dubansky, L. S., & Chin, M. L. Intensive care in adolescent pregnancy. *Obstetrics Gynecology,* 1978, *52,* 179–188.

Shah, F., Zelnick, M., & Kantner, J. F. Unprotected intercourse among unwed teenagers. *Family Planning Perspectives,* 1975, *7,* 39–44.

Sorenson, R. C. *Adolescent sexuality in contemporary America.* New York: World, 1972.

Zelnick, M., & Kantner, J. F. Sexual and contraceptive experience of young unmarried women in the United States, 1976 and 1971. *Family Planning Perspectives,* 1977, *9,* 55–77.

Zelnick, M., & Kantner, J.F.,Contraceptive patterns and premarital pregnancy among women aged 15–19 in 1976. *Family Planning Perspectives,* 1978, *10,* 135–142.

chapter 5

LATER PREGNANCY

Alice Eichholz
Joan Offerman-Zuckerberg

Pregnancy is a life crisis, a time when a woman's identity is challenged and likely changed. As such, it contains all of the ambivalences, fears, anxieties, and victorious feelings attached to life crises and their resolutions. Pregnancy after the age of 35, involves, moreover, responding to the physical and psychological impact of aging.

Today many women have spent 15 to 20 years developing a career and reach the age of 35 with different attitudes and feelings toward becoming pregnant and childrearing than were present during their younger years. This chapter considers the physical and psychological aspects of participating in that part of being a woman which has previously been set aside, ambivalently pursued, or denied. From our own research, clinical observations and interviews with women, we have observed several issues which may be applicable to understanding the psychology of pregnancy in women over 35.

The physical components of aging do play some part in the process. Intrapsychic needs, such as the wish to reproduce and nurture the next generation also are involved. While the issues are complicated, we have considered the problem only as it relates to the married woman who has chosen to have the baby. Some of the psychological factors to be discussed transcend chronological age. The discussion of these factors will focus upon older women and how they experience these dimensions of becoming and being pregnant.

One crucial psychological difference between women who have babies in their 20's and young 30's and women who delay pregnancy until after 35 is found in the degree and process of *separation* from their mothers. The decision to become or continue a pregnancy is rooted in a woman's relationship with her mother. From her mother's unconscious and conscious attitudes, wishes, and experiences, a woman derives and then recreates her own attitudes toward pregnancy. Because the oedipal issues of "stepping into your mother's shoes" reemerge during the developmental stages of pregnancy and childbirth, the older woman has more likely worked through the major impact of these issues. An older woman might have surpassed her own mother in many ways and has experienced and resolved some of the ambivalent wishes associated with those accomplishments. Such resolutions have resulted from work accomplishments or social relationships. Consequently, the woman over 35 may often make clearer, more mature choices regarding pregnancy and childrearing, than would have been possible for her at an earlier time. This process and the effects of *individuation* also may mean that she recognizes herself as separate from her new baby and growing child. LeBoyer (1975) interestingly observes that a major difference in the mother's ability to accept the process of separation in birth can be observed in her ability to say, "I am a mother," rather than "this is my child." The older woman is more likely to have fulfilled large parts of herself in terms of her life's goals and less likely to ask a child to do that for her. In contrast, a younger woman, particularly a teenager, may have a tendency to use the pregnancy as a way of trying to fulfill herself and/or to state independence from her mother, rather than having worked through her own separateness.

Unfortunately, it is still difficult for a woman to find a sense of fulfillment in our culture in ways other than by having children. Consequently, it has been psychologically difficult for women to see themselves as complex individuals with needs, hopes, and attitudes separate from their mother's expectations. However, the recent popularity of books like Nancy Friday's *My Mother, My Self* (1977) suggests that today's women desire to address themselves to the process of separation in a way that was very difficult to do so before. Being separate is not just doing something different, but experiencing yourself with an independent psychic life apart from your mother and the decisions she made with her life.

While older women may be more individuated and therefore more psychologically capable of being "good enough mothers," they may find it harder to engage and empathize with a child's needs and demands simply because they are further away from the chronological experience of childhood. Many older women state that because they had an investment in the adult world, they felt it was harder to adapt to service a baby's demands, but that they also felt more psychologically informed and aware of the need to meet those demands than they would have been at a younger age.

The distinction is clearly the ability to be rooted securely enough in yourself in order to empathize with your baby and yet not unconsciously overidentify, or see the child as an excessive, narcisstic extension of yourself. It would not be surprising to find that older mothers of first children spend less time with their own infants because they are more invested in the adult world, but that the quality of time might be more meaningful and free of conflict. However, some older women express that having a child permits a welcome relief from the adult world and enjoy the delicious protectiveness of being at home, and not having to contend with the environmental consequences and daily political arenas of the adult world. Perhaps for these older women childbearing becomes a concrete way to change one's life-style and restate identity.

In addition to separation phenomena, *ambivalence* can be a part of the nature of being a mother. We have not developed sufficiently enough as a culture or as individuals to make easy decisions about ourselves in relationship to our children. Jane Lazarre in *The Mother Knot* (1975) looks at one woman's struggle with the ambivalences that have been part of being a mother. From a more theoretical point of view, Heffner (1978) suggests that

> psychoanalysis has imposed on mothers the responsibility of raising emotionally healthy children, but did not help them achieve this goal without leaving them with excessive guilt and feelings of inadequacy. The women's movement responded to that plight by attempting to liberate women from the mothering role but has not helped them become successful with it (p. vii).

Many mothers feel an active conflict between their needs and the child's demands. Often this is expressed in the older woman in ambivalence about staying home with an infant or leaving a career temporarily. A younger woman, who first has children and then begins work on a career outside of the home may not feel the conflict in the same way, or possibly as acutely.

She has to contend, however, with problems of establishing herself in a career and competing with younger women as well as with men.

A third psychological aspect that differentiates the older mother from the younger one is *the ability to accept and to mourn loss.* Involved in the process of mourning and grief is the capacity to hold on and let go. There is probably no more powerful psychological preparation for dealing with children's growth and development than this ability. A woman over 35 has been through more attachments and separations, simply because of her age. At a younger age, a mother may have the feeling that the child needs her totally when in reality it is often the mother herself who totally needs the child. Age has a way of helping to establish limits on our desparate attempts at total symbiosis and may allow a person to see oneself and others more distinctly. Because of this, the same people may do better at parenting later than if they had made the choice at a younger age.

The last psychological issue being considered involves the psychological and physical aspects of later, first pregnancies. To many people, "over 35" means that your cup is half empty, i.e. half of your life gone, as opposed to half of your life left to live. The half empty cup analogy can play havoc with the decision to become pregnant. Women reach this age where the culture, superstition, and folklore convey that pregnancy will result in damaged children, and possible fetal and/or maternal death. While in the last few years these superstitions have been challenged and changed, the underlying fears are often present in the woman's decision as to when to have children. Some even consider pregnancy after 35 as a confrontation to cultural norms.

Age 35 and up often is the time when a woman is depicted as a temptress—safe, unfertile ground for sexual fantasies and practices. Unfortunately, these attitudes about the process of aging in relationship to physical abilities and sexuality are also apparent in the medical professions' response to later pregnancies. Some gynecologists express this attitude in comments like: "you don't have much time left," "if you don't do something soon, there'll be no chances left," and "if you are too old, your body won't function properly and it will be dangerous." While there is an element of reality in these comments, they alone are not helpful in allowing a woman to come to terms with her own individual psychological and physical concerns regarding pregnancy. The wise doctor is able to help a woman evaluate her specific situation in a way that makes the decision less of a threat than "last chance" attempts.

The medical profession's attitudes about pregnancy after 35 ranges from those who consider all first pregnancies after 35 high risk to the view that *age alone* should not be considered a factor in high-risk pregnancies. In some hospitals, the older primipara is scheduled automatically for a Cesarean section with the justification that her body will not function the way a younger woman's will. One gynecologist, for example, reported that a 42-year-old woman, in labor for the first time had been prepared for a cesarean section with the obstretrics team waiting for his arrival to perform the surgery. Until he arrived and was able to rectify the situation, no one had checked to determine whether or not the operation was indeed necessary. The woman was progressing very well and actively engaged in labor with every indication that she could deliver the child without surgical intervention, which she did.

Among the numerous books and articles on the genetic aspects of later pregnancies are Apgar & Beck, 1972; Mc Cauley, 1976; and Price, 1977. Rheingold (1964, 1967) suggests that the sources of damaged child fantasies appear to be rooted in a woman's prejudice toward her failing or failed femininity. It may also be in her injured narcissism related to the natural process of aging. What is important to the woman over 35 is that the statistics appear to make her fears much more of a reality. The "what if" becomes "more possible" or so she thinks. While the statistics usually quoted seem frightening, initially, they need to be evaluated with a critical eye. Is it only age which is the variable or are other factors also tested? Does the research apply to the ovum or also to the sperm which participated in creating the new life? Because these are important questions for medical research to answer, present results have to be considered inconclusive. In Down's syndrome babies, for example, it appears that age of the mother is the sole factor. However, more Down's syndrome babies are born to mothers *under* 35 than to mothers over 35 simply because more babies in general are born to mothers under 35. While the percentage of Down's syndrome babies rises sharply in women over 40, the fertility rate also has declined and rarely are factors such as nutrition, and other high-risk variables considered. The effects of other contributing variables rarely reach popular understanding.

What the woman over 35 needs to consider when deciding whether or not to become pregnant is whether she feels physically and psychologically capable of meeting the life challenges and changes that pregnancy brings. A good physician will be able to help her to evaluate the physical dimension without using statistics or veiled threats and generalizations that are not particularly helpful. The medical specialist can help her to evaluate her own risks, based upon her history and needs, and not those of the general population. Ideally, if mental health workers, gynecologists, and midwives worked together, a woman would be able to explore both the physical and psychological aspects of the decision with professional help.

Many physicians routinely recommend amniocentesis, a medical procedure which determines whether the amniotic fluid surrounding the fetus is normal, for women over 40 years of age. Discolored or contaminated fluid indicates the presence of irregularities or physical deformities in the fetus. Many major chromosonal defects such as Down's syndrome; metabolic and biochemical disorders such as Tay-Sachs; sex-related conditions such as hemophilia; and disorders of the spine or nervous system such as spina bifida can be detected by this procedure. The fluid will also reveal the sex of the child. This procedure can be seen as an advancement in dealing with the anxieties produced from concerns over the baby's normality.

However, the procedure and its physical and psychological consequences are not without potential risk. To determine the position of the fetus and umbilical cord and to help direct the insertion of the long needle through the woman's abdomen sonar (ultrahigh sound waves) is used. Its safety has been questioned.

The amniocentesis is usually done in the 4th month of pregnancy (most frequently in the 15th to 17th week) and the amniotic fluid is then put through 2 to 3 weeks of laboratory analysis before the test results are available. (This would allow for sufficient time to perform a therapeutic abortion if the fetus is found to be defective.) The psychological results of the test should be considered in determining whether or not to use the procedure to alleviate fears of producing a damaged child. Waiting 3 weeks in the middle of a pregnancy for such test results can have traumatic effects on the woman and couple. If it were possible to speed the results of the test some of this anxiety would be lessened. Also very important is the loss of fantasy about the sex of the baby after the test results have been received (although some parents specifically request not to be given that information). Knowledge about the sex of the child might in some cases obscure healthy anxiety and preparation for the new baby.

Finally, some existential differences between younger and older women also may have some impact on adjustment to late pregnancy. The older woman has waited a long time, and, as long as she does not put all her hopes and dreams on the child, the child will most likely have more value to her. The child who is both consciously and unconsciously wanted will be happier and easier to care for and to parent. In addition, because of the value of the child to the woman who has waited, she is less likely to be concerned about the child's sex simply because having a healthy child is most important. With fewer expectations related to sex, there is likely to be a more tolerant attitude when the child seeks his or her identity.

All of the foregoing aspects have some relationship to problems with separation, probably one of the most difficult areas to resolve in growing up. The goals for any professional working with a pregnant woman, regardless of her age, need to include developing tolerance for a certain amount of ambivalence, developing a capacity to accept and mourn loss, and forming a sense of self separate from that of her mother. For all women, the ability to empathize with a child to accept the support offered by significant others without becoming alienated or a childlike nonparticipant are important to deal with the psychological and physical upheaval of pregnancy. For psychologists such goals are not unfamiliar. All professionals, however, could consider these goals in helping each woman accept the challenge and change of pregnancy and childbirth.

REFERENCES

Apgar, V., & Beck, J. *Is my baby all right?* New York: Trident Press, 1972.

Friday, N. *My mother, my self.* New York: Delacorte Press, 1977.

Heffner, E. *Mothering: The emotional experience of motherhood after Freud and feminism.* New York: Doubleday, 1978.

Lazarre, J. *The mother knot.* New York: McGraw-Hill, 1975.

Leboyee, F. *Birth without violence.* New York: Knopf, 1975.

McCauley, C. S. *Pregnancy after thirty-five.* New York: Dutton, 1976.

Price, J. *You're not too old to have a baby.* New York: Farrar, Straus, Giroux, 1977.

Rheingold, J. *The fear of being a woman: A theory of maternal destructiveness.* New York: Grune & Stratton, 1964.

Rheingold, J. *Mother, anxiety and death.* Boston: Little Brown, 1967.

chapter 6

SINGLE WOMEN WHO ELECT TO BEAR A CHILD

Phima Engelstein,
Maxine Antell-Buckley,
Phyllis Urman-Klein

The literature on the unmarried mother (Barglow et al., 1968; Bernard, 1944; Catell, 1954; Horn, 1976; Kasanin & Handschin, 1941; Roberts, 1966; Vincent, 1962; Young, 1954) has been based predominantly on the study of the pregnant women who come to the attention of foundling hospitals or homes for unwed mothers. These, however, constitute a small fraction of the total population of unwed mothers. To what degree the unwed older mother, who can maintain herself without recourse to an agency, resembles the younger woman who does make agency contact is not clear. The few studies that do in passing refer to the older professional single mother, and these are also based on women who contact agencies, stress her immaturity and her psychological pathology.

We decided to study a small group of older, middle-class

This project was funded by a grant from the Society for the Psychological Study of Social Issues.

women, who planned to bear children out of marriage and who had not come to the attention of a psychiatric agency. We expected that the fact that these women were older and had chosen their motherhood consciously would significantly set them apart from the younger group of mothers, despite possible similarity in dynamics and motivation. We were also prepared for the possibility that in the present social climate their choice might represent strength and the courage to take a radical stance rather than pathology.

SUBJECTS

Our sample consisted of the first eight women who volunteered for the study in response to advertisements in college or local newspapers or on hearing about our study from friends. All were white and unmarried; all had professions and careers at which they were employed; two had returned to school. They ranged in age from 25 to 38; most were 30 to 35. At initial contact, two were pregnant and six had children under 4 years of age. This was the first child for all. Half of the women had at one time been married, but these marriages had terminated in divorce after a few months or a few years. None of the pregnancies were conceived while the women were married. When seen, each was living alone, except for the two who shared households with the father of their child.

They did not come from broken or economically disadvantaged homes. Not one was herself illegitimate or had a mother who was promiscuous. Three were Jewish, three Protestant, and two Catholic. They were not active politically, but with one exception described themselves as liberal or radical in outlook. None was avowedly homosexual. In short, these women were productive, active members of society, who had achieved scholastically, held responsible positions, and lived largely within socially acceptable norms.

METHOD

The data were obtained through taped clinical interviews conducted jointly by the authors, psychological testing on six of the subjects who agreed to it, and self-administered family and sexual history questionnaires devised for the study. The two women pregnant on initial contact were interviewed once during the pregnancy and again postpartum, the others only once.

RESULTS

The small number and self-selected nature of the sample raise questions as to how general the findings are, but we think the striking similarities we found are worth reporting. The subjects will be described as a group rather than through individual case histories, partly for reasons of confidentiality.

Families of Origin

Our subjects were either the oldest children or the first-born daughters. All of them grew up in two-parent families which were, however, disrupted in four of the eight cases by the death of one or both of the parents during the subject's adolescence or young adulthood.

The parental marriages, described as "bitter, incompatible, violent," were either intensely and openly conflictual or characterized by simmering tension and bickering which erupted periodically into open conflict. One subject said, "I do not know how my mother and father survived." In addition, all eight of the marriages were described as singularly lacking in closeness and open expression of affection. The parents were unavailable to each other as well as to their children; each was left to deal with her problems alone. The children grew up feeling painfully lonely. "There was not and still is not emotional support in the family," one subject noted.

Most of the fathers were depicted as depressed men who were disappointed in life. Although only one father was actually hospitalized for depression late in life, and another was in fact old, deaf, and sickly, many of these men were unconsciously perceived by their daughters as worn out, passive, ineffectual, and emotionally unavailable.

Paradoxically, a number of women described themselves as their father's favorites, or as closest to him of all the children. Feeling that their fathers wished them to be boys, some of the women tried to be sons to their fathers and were drawn to activities and interests which they could share with the fathers. But they all described the fathers' attitudes to them as containing an important element of disparagement and devaluation. They complained of being made to feel "stupid, inferior, helpless." One subject summarized this ambivalent relationship by saying her father made her feel "both very special and very incompetent." Thus, encouragement and transient availability alternated with withdrawal of support and criticism.

Our subjects saw their mothers as dependent and intensely unhappy women whose efforts to engage their emotionally unavailable mates proved largely ineffectual. All were experienced by their daughters as lacking in tenderness; either as unavailable and ungiving, or as unempathic and intrusive in their giving, i.e., "obiligatory mothers." They conveyed the impression that they felt too burdened to be imposed upon for love or affection. Instead, the mothers turned to their daughters for mothering, for protection against their husbands, and to defend against their fears of abandonment and depression. The children felt emotionally unsupported and alone except when they gratified their mothers' need to be mothered. "I always approached my mother as my child because I always had to protect her."

Their mothers' unhappiness seems to have been experienced by these young girls as a demand that they relieve their mothers of their burdens, mother and protect them, and thus assure their survival. A number of our subjects unconsciously perceived leaving or separating from their mothers as equivalent to death. (Interestingly, the mother of one subject did, indeed, suffer her first acute, and fatal, asthmatic attack when our subject left on a trip to Europe.) The mothers used withdrawal of emotional supplies as a way of discouraging steps toward individuation. Conversely, through their overvaluation of their daughters as "the most important thing in their lives" the mothers reinforced the notion that the children were essential to their survival, thereby promoting the grandiosity as well as the dependency of their daughters. In some cases, the mother expressly stated her expectation that the daughter never marry but remain in the family to care for her and the children. Four of the subjects actually took on the function of parenting younger siblings. Though they resented these responsibilities, they also welcomed them because mothering gratified their need for closeness and reduced their loneliness. Thus, our women were from an early age identified as little mothers in their families, and they internalized this attribution in a core identification. The idea of a child as potentially life saving was also internalized.

In short, although our women did not describe gross maternal rejection, and did not come from disorganized homes, they seemed, much like the young mothers described by Bernard (1944), to have received "too little parental love, protection, esteem, encouragement and support ... to develop emotional security."

Object Relations

The object relations of this group of women are characterized by great interpersonal anxiety in a context of great object need. On a conscious level, most reported feeling an intense and lifelong loneliness and difficulties in making "close loving ties." For many of the women, this loneliness ceased for the first time on becoming pregnant. The fetus became their longed-for companion.

Close relationships for them are infused with anxiety for many reasons. Perhaps the foremost among these is the fear that in intimate relationships the individual is in danger of being controlled and forced to become an extension of the other, as in their early relationships with their mothers, or abandoned, as in their relationships with their fathers. These expectations are in part a projection of their own oral-dependent needs and of unconscious yearnings for an object who will be totally attuned to them and with whom they can fuse. The yearning for fusion with another object as a way of avoiding the aloneness of separateness and to repair their empty, devalued, and damaged self-images is expressed beautifully in a Rorschach percept of one subject: "The two parts have the makings of one person."

Sexual Identity

The sexual identity of our subjects appeared to be characterized by a confused combination of bisexual elements, disparagement of both male and female as flawed and castrated, a splitting of sexual and maternal elements, and a condensation of genital and pregenital aims. Evidence of unresolved bisexuality abounded in the psychological data, notably in, such Rorschach percepts as: "It's either a man's testicles or a woman's labia," or "the faces look like men but they have bosoms," or "a pregnant man." It was also reflected in the acknowledged homosexual fantasies, dreams, or overt experiences of most of the subjects. It probably also contributed to the interest of some of the subjects in group sex and the predilection of others to friendships and, in one case, marriage with homosexual men.

The unconscious equation of femaleness with incompleteness and inferiority was pervasive and not modified by the contradictory attribution to women of a kind of strength and wild rebellious power, which emerged as a minor theme. The projected male images were likewise flawed and weak; understandably, the attempts of our women to compensate for their sense of inferiority through phallic, paternal identifications were not stable. However, though men were seen as essentially weak and themselves in need of nuturance, their sexuality was perceived as intensely aggressive, so that the women experienced intense fears of phallic intrusion.

The feminine identity of these women became organized around their early mothering identifications from which sexual and erotic elements were split off. In this, our women seemed to illustrate one type of identification with the mother which Deutsch (1933) has described as follows: "the idea of having a child is acceptable and only the part of the man as a sexual partner is denied. The girl wants to be a mother and to have a child, but quite by herself, by immaculate conception or parthenogenesis." The compulsive desire for a child served the function of confirming their femininity and reconciling them to their bodies. On the other hand, their insistence on having the child without a co-parent expressed an unconscious grandiose fantasy that they were both male and female.

Relationship to the Father

The literature on the relationship of the unwed mother to the biological father of the child is, with few exceptions, in agreement with Kasanin and Handschin's (1941) formulation: "The men responsible for her pregnancies did not exist for her as such, but were phantom fathers through the mediums of which she was able to act out an unresolved oedipal situation."

While it is also true of our women that their choice of men was determined largely by unresolved oedipal issues, it needs to be emphasized that in contrast to the younger unwed mothers, our women *were* for the most part emotionally involved with their men in intense relationships, some of which had lasted for years. The chosen lovers resembled the fathers in significant ways and were in some cases consciously identified by the women with their fathers or with their younger brothers. In other ways, they were unacceptable, even forbidden, choices because of their race, religion, social class, or age.

The timing of the decision to become pregnant derived in most cases from the woman's fear that the relationship would not endure or the perception that it was in fact already in the process of dissolution. Thus, the pregnancy represented the unconscious acknowledgement that the relationship was not viable despite the wish that it continue. While some of the women fantasized that once pregnant, they might bring the man around to marriage, they largely knew this was unrealistic. Some even acknowledged knowing that becoming pregnant might hasten and assure losing the man.

All but two of the women became pregnant without informing the fathers of their intention to conceive, and notified the men of their pregnancies, if at all, when it was too late to abort. Two women shared their intention beforehand, the same two who were still living with their men after the children were born. With three exceptions, the men were noticeably uninvolved in supporting the women during the pregnancy and delivery or thereafter. While four of the women felt that it was important for the child to know his father and to maintain some contact with him, only the two who were living with the father allowed this to happen. But even these two made it clear that the man's access to the child was contingent on the mother's retaining control.

It would seem, then, that unresolved oedipal issues determined the choice of men for these women, but that their guilt about oedipal wishes led them to look for men who would be unavailable and disappointing. In this context, the baby conceived with these men became a restitution for the impending, half-acquiesced-in loss of the forbidden love object. Through the child, the woman maintained a symbolic connection with the absent father/husband, though she took care to exclude her offspring from a real connection with him.

But the renunciation of the lover/father implicit in the decision to become pregnant by men who were not going to be permanent mates and coparents was also welcome for reasons other than oedipal guilt. First, it fostered the omnipotent fantasy that the child was the woman's own doing and tended to obscure the fact that the man had anything to do with it. Second, their act was a settling of scores with their fathers whom they had experienced as unavailable and unreliable. Third, the need to feel in total control of her life and in particular of her child was another reason for banishing the father/husband from a mother/child dyad. A number of women expressed fear of a father's power to take the child away from a mother. One woman said, "I was jealous about the baby before she was even conceived . . . I had fantasies of conceiving and then disappearing without telling the father. I certainly did not want to get married. I didn't want the father to have any legal possibility of taking the baby away from me. I'm not going to let anyone take her away from me until she's old enough to go on her own."

Decision

Many of the women "knew" early that they would not marry but that they wanted a child. To the question, "When did you first decide to have a child?" a number answered, "A long time ago, as well as more recently" or "I have always wanted a child." Some recalled being sufficiently preoccupied with the wish to have a child during their high school years as to have discussed with their mothers the possibility of having one out of wedlock at that time. In explaining why she decided to have a child, one woman said, "In the deepest part of me I was a mother. I needed a child to complete me, to take care of. I always treated other people as my children."

Although the wish for a child was a lifelong preoccupation, the actual decision to become pregnant was preceded in adulthood for the majority of our sample by a period of time, often extending for several years, during which the women experienced their wish to mother with renewed intensity and set about to prepare for motherhood. Under the pressure of realizing that their biological time for having a baby was running out, the women seem to have moved in two directions: on the one hand, a renewed search for a mate; and on the other, a series of preparations intended to equip them for the task of mothering on their own. This period of preparation marked a consolidation of their personal and professional lives. For some, this meant securing their professional status, assuring a steady income and some savings, obtaining adequate living space and last, the physical readying of their bodies. In the case of two women concerned with the possibility of sterility, this last extended to "trial" pregnancies, unconsciously desired to test out if they could conceive, and which were then aborted. One woman gave up smoking; another lost 25 pounds. For two of the women, however, this period is best described as a time of confusion and becoming pregnant as an effort at staving off disorganization.

The psychological consolidation and professional success of most of the women were, however, colored by restlessness and a general dissatisfaction, a feeling of lack of fulfillment or futility in work, and a longing for something more satisfying. "I had to make a radical change in my life," said one. "I wanted a greater commitment in my life," said another.

It was in this context of dissatisfaction despite consolidation or confusion due to a loss of direction that an impending or actual object loss resonated with the underlying intense loneliness and depression and provided the final push in the decision to have a baby. Greenberg et al. (1959), Loesch & Greenberg (1962), Heiman & Levitt (1960), Blos (1957), Gedo (1965), and others have pointed to important object losses followed by depressive reactions as among the significant events in the life situations of unmarried women who became pregnant, and our data amply confirm this observation. In our sample, significant events preceding pregnancy included multiple losses of important people through separation or death and the dissolution of significant heterosexual relationships. These were experienced as narcissistic injuries as well as loses and triggered anxiety and depression.

Despite the conscious readying for motherhood, the conception for half our women was described by them as, "not a total accident, but also not planned." This meant that at a certain point the woman stopped using contraception but did not acknowledge to herself that she intended to conceive. Rather, she felt that the conception was left to fate. For the other half of the group, the decision to conceive was conscious and deliberate. Thus, for example, one woman selectively did not use contraception with the man she had chosen to be the father of her child, while using it in other sexual encounters.

The need of half the women to obscure to themselves the intention to conceive is striking. It suggests guilt around the acting out of a forbidden wish. Guilt about exploiting an unwilling or unknowing man may also have been involved in making fate a partner in the decision. Once pregnant, many struggled with the decision to keep the pregnancy. Their initial reaction on finding themselves pregnant was a mixture of pride and relief in their ability to conceive, but also a last hesitation about the wisdom of the enterprise. All but one reported considering abortion. All sought confirmation of their decision to keep the baby from someone important to them. But they tended to accept only encouragement and to ignore disapproving or cautionary counsel. While six of the eight eventually apprised the biological father of the pregnancy, they did so only after prior discussion with friends, family, or priest, and after it was too late to consider abortion.

DISCUSSION

The fantasy of having a baby, that is, of becoming a mother, which perhaps in every girl stems as much from an effort to find a substitute for the mother who separated from her as out of a wish to obtain something from father that would compensate her for the realization that she is without a penis, had in the case of our women a particular intensity. First, given their mothers' singular inability to be empathic and affectionate, the daughters felt uniquely deprived and abandoned; this led to a lifelong search for a constant, loving object. Second, the mothers' failure to satisfy their daughters' need for dependency created a tendency for the daughters to look to the fathers not only for support against their controlling and narcissistically involving mothers but for the very mothering they had missed. This found some resonance in the fathers' own unmet needs for mothering and resulted in an infusion of strong preoedipal longings into the oedipal realtionship. These longings suffered renewed frustration due to the fathers' depressive withdrawal, which reinforced the daughters' need for a substitute object. Third, the perception that the bond between their parents was flawed gave a particular strength as well as danger to the oedipal longings of the girls.

Thus, their wish for a baby contained many elements: identification with the mother; the wish for an object with whom they could duplicate a mother/child bond, but in which they would be the controlling rather than the controlled; the wish to replace mother in the father's affection; and the wish to get something from the father.

In late adolescence, the wish for a child reemerged in many of our subjects with renewed strength. According to Helene Deutsch (1945), "The task of adolescence is not only to master the Oedipus complex, but also to continue the work begun during pre-puberty, that is, to give adult forms to the old, much deeper and much more primitive ties with the mother, and to end all bisexual wavering in favor of a definite heterosexual orientation." It is precisely at this crucial developmental point that many of our women became obsessed with the idea of motherhood. In circumstances where other young women are filled with romantic fantasies toward some male figure, or actually fall in love, these women experienced a revival of the girlish wish to have a child. This wish reflected a developmental faltering, an inability to make a shift of libidinal investment from pregenital to genital love objects and from familial objects to those outside the family. The wish to mother, divorced as it was from a relationship with a male and appearing in place of it, implied a regressive wish to hold on to a mother/child relationship instead of moving on to mature genital functioning and a relationship with a mate. In addition, the consolidation of identity around being a mother, a nurturer, rather than a heterosexual mate, represented an attempt to avoid a decisive separation from the parents through a defensive partial identification with both parents in which the maternal and paternal aspects are emphasized while the sexual and erotic elements are split off and kept hidden. Thus, the sexual and erotic aspects of the woman's femininity remain unintegrated with the maternal elements that were precociously and defensively elaborated in the fantasy life of the girl. As a result, bisexual wavering is not resolved, and the Oedipus complex is not mastered. Pregenital drives remain central.

But while the fantasy of bearing a child represents a clinging to childhood objects, it can also be seen as a defense against the danger of attaching the reawakened pregenital and newly emergent genital urges to infantile objects. The fantasied child may be thought of as a transitional object representing a fused father/mother of childhood, but containing also *in statu nascendi* a new object, neither parent nor self nor quite other. As such, it represents a compromise between a narcissistic and more mature, differentiated object. Its function is to facilitate the adolescent's detachment from incestuous objects, to dimish the experience of depression associated with that loss, and to allay the anxiety engendered around making new attachments. It is noteworthy, however, that the child fantasy was already in adolescence associated for many of the women with an awareness that the wish for a child was not likely for them to be realized in marriage. The association of the child fantasy

with an out-of-wedlock state reflected the fact that a noninces-
tuous object choice could not be made. Hence, the fantasy of
procreation had to be divorced from the context of marriage.

We speculate that the very elaboration of such a child
fantasy may have had a role in enabling these women to proceed
with their developmental tasks and averted the need to act it out
in adolescence. In fact, many of our women did go on to physical separation from their families, pursuit of educational objectives, involvement in career, heterosexual relationships, and
even marriage in some cases. In this they can be contrasted with
the younger illegitimate mothers who, having similar developmental liabilities in respect to faulty separation from insufficiently loving and unempathic parents and fixation on oral level
satisfactions, *do* become pregnant at this point, short-circuiting
development in a more drastic fashion.

The eventual decision to act on their wish seems to have
been determined for a majority of our sample by a combination
of factors: the realization that they were reaching the biological
limits of safe childbearing; acknowledgement of the fact that
they were unable or unwilling to sustain a long-term relationship with a man; discontent with work; loss of an important
relationship; a conviction that they could financially support
such a venture without incurring social condemnation; and
finally, the fantasy that a child would provide them with a
loving object that would revitalize their lives and assuage their
loneliness.

The dissolution of a romantic relationship or some other
loss, which preceded conception in all cases, seems to have
activated earlier separation anxiety and depression, and reawakened a regressive yearning to recreate the fused union with
the mother. The wish to become pregnant, a compromise formation between the wish to regress and be mothered and a
defense against regression through mothering, reemerged
strongly, and this time was acted upon.

Conclusions

Becoming a mother for the women in our sample is not an accidental or impulsive act but the final realization of an essential aspect of their identity and the attempted gratification of their lifelong yearning for the good preoedipal mother. Given the fact that our subjects do not differ with respect to motivation for motherhood, personality organization, or pathology from some women who marry in order to have children, one might wonder why our women did not marry to have a child or why they did not bear children when they were married. We suspect that what is special about our women is their fear of marriage. This has its conscious roots in their rejection of the kind of lonely, conflictful, and unaffectionate relationships that existed in their parents' marriages. Unconsciously, a close relationship with an adult mobilizes their dependency needs and regressive yearnings for fusion with a maternal figure. These yearnings are feared because they threaten a lifelong accommodation of pseudoindependence and imply the threat of being controlled or exploited or abandoned in such a relationship. Second, our women's wish for a child is grounded in their need for an object who will be a constant and exclusive object for them; one whom they can control. The husband/father is perceived by the women as threatening the mother's exclusive control of the child. Third, marriage would undermine the defensive splitting of maternal and sexual roles necessitated by their unresolved infantile attachments and negative identifications with their mothers. Last, competition with both parents finds expression in the need to prove that, unlike their mothers, they have the courage to raise a child without a husband, thereby showing the man that he is not needed.

The consequence of single motherhood for our women appears as of now at least to have been more adaptive than destructive. Social position and professional standing have been maintained by and large. The women have not withdrawn from work or friendships in favor of absorption with the child. Some have repaired their relationships with their mothers. Whether or not the child will protect them from depression in the long run is unknown. At present all report feeling much less lonely and more purposeful and fulfilled. Some even speak of having a second child.

We recognize that the women have an investment in emphasizing the positive outcome of their choice and that these assertions must therefore be viewed with caution. The long-term effect on their lives as well as on the development of their offspring remains to be studied. Can they avoid repeating with their children the exploitation they suffered at the hands of their mothers?

REFERENCES

Barglow, P., Bornstein, M., Exum, D. B., Wright, M. K., & Bisotsky, H. M. Some psychiatric aspects of illegitimate pregnancy in early adolescence. *American Journal of Orthopsychiatry,* 1968, *38,* 672–687.

Bernard, V. Psychodynamics of unmarried motherhood in early adolescence. *Nervous Child,* 1944, *4,* 26–45.

Blos, P. Preoedipal factors in the etiology of female delinquency. *Psychoanalytic Study of the Child,* 1957, *12,* 229–249.

Cattell, J. Psychodynamic & clinical observations in a group of unmarried mothers. *American Journal of Psychiatry,* 1964, *3,* 337–342.

Deutsch, H. Motherhood and sexuality. *Psychoanalytic. Quarterly,* 1933, *2,* 476–488.

Deutsch, H. *Psychology of women.* New York: Grune & Stratton, 1945.

Gedo, J. E. Unmarried motherhood. A paradigmatic single case study. *International Journal of Psychoanalysis,* 1965, *46,* 352–357.

Greenberg, N. H., Loesch, J. G., & Laken, M. Life situations associated with the onset of pregnancy. *Psychosomatic Medicine,* 1959, *21,* 296–310.

Heiman, M., & Levitt, E. The role of separation and depression in out-of-wedlock pregnancy. *American Journal of Orthopsychiatry,* 1960, *30,* 166–174.

Horn, J. M., & Turner R. G. Minnesota multiphasic personality inventory profiles among subgroups of unwed mothers. *Journal Consulting and Clinical Psychology,* 1976, *44,* 25–33.

Kasanin, J., & Handschin, S., Psychodynamic factors in illegitimacy. *American Journal of Orthopsychiatry,* 1941, *11.* 66–84.

Loesch, J., & Greenberg, N. Some scientific areas of conflicts observed during pregnancy: A comparative study of married and unmarried pregnant women. *American Journal of Orthopsychiatry,* 1962, *32,* 624–636.

Roberts, R. W. *The unwed mother.* New York: Harper & Row, 1966.

Vincent, C. *Unmarried motherhood,* Glencoe, Ill.: Free Press, 1962.

Young, L. *Out of wedlock.* New York: McGraw-Hill, 1954.

chapter 7

PONDERING PARENTHOOD
Issues Facing Couples
Deciding To Parent

Amy Miller-Cohen

Probably one of the most significant decisions made by contemporary couples is whether or not to bear and rear children. This chapter focuses upon factors affecting this decision. The role and effects of professional intervention in the decision-making process are discussed for couples contemplating a first child.

Recently, articles in popular magazines (e.g. Cizmar, 1979; Dreifus, 1977) have pointed to the difficulties some couples have in making the parenting decision. In the past, many, if not most, couples did not make the childbearing decision consciously and jointly. Today, however, because of advances in birth control, it is actually difficult for people to avoid consciously making some childbearing choices. Ory (1978) has speculated that now more young couples than ever before discuss parenthood and make childbearing decisions prior to marriage commitments, and that this trend is increasing.

Much appreciation is felt for the partnership for Dr. Robert D. Cohen in working with the couples.

In this era of dual-career marriages, high divorce rates, and economic inflation, many couples are keenly aware of the negative aspects of being parents. As Radl (1973) states, these negative aspects and attitudes need to be explored. As Peck (1971) has suggested, however, there also are oppressive forces in our culture *for* having children. Bernard (1974), relating motherhood to womanhood, states "the true choice for all women with respect to motherhood will not be a reality until the enormous pressures on women to make them want children are abated" (p. 42). Although birth control technically allows couples to consciously choose to have a child, adequate support for other life choices, including nonparenthood or full-time involvement of a woman in a career, is necessary for couples to really feel free to consider parenthood as a choice. The many "accidents" from which children of birth control users are born suggests that unconscious determinants, some affected by external pressures, are involved in the decision to become parents.

Boynton's (1978) research on identity development and attitudes toward motherhood in young professional women suggests a developmental sequence for making such decisions. First, women resolve their polarizations about motherhood and conflicts about their own mothers. Then, their relationships with their husbands and with their own careers need to be considered.

Veevers (1973, 1975) found that when people lean toward nonparenthood, they avoid spending time with peers who do have children. She noted that couples who did not decide on parenthood prior to marriage tended to come to the decision as a series of postponments. After many delays, age (McCauley, 1976; Nortman, 1974) necessarily became a significant consideration.

Ravich (1978) suggested that the act of making decisions regarding potential parenthood can result in conflict, stress, and interspouse testing. Others also have suggested that if parenthood is linked with maturity and adulthood additional intra- and interpersonal stress will result.

Two self-help books are detailed in giving factors to consider. Whelan (1975) can be credited with the first comprehensive treatment of the "baby question." She states that there are parent and nonparent aspects in everyone and spells out the rational and irrational components in the decision-making process. Her work is based on interviews with parents, nonparents, and mental health professionals. *Ourselves and Our Children* (1978) devotes a chapter to exploring thoughts on whether to choose to parent. Many couples have sought professional help in their attempts to make their decisions regarding childbearing.

Workshops and Counseling Sessions

In light of the above considerations, the author and her husband conducted workshops and held counseling sessions specifically for couples attempting to decide whether or not to have a first child. The decision to have children involves more than a decision for pregnancy and childbirth; it is a decision to become a parent as well. The workshops, therefore, were entitled "Pondering Parenthood."

Five principles guided our work. The first is that *the parenting decision is a couple decision,* although each spouse does bring his and her own motives to the decision. Thus, the decision to have a child ought not to be seen as the domain of the woman or of the woman and her doctor or midwife, but as that of a man and woman together. The second principle is based on the observation that increasing numbers of men and women have, for one reason or another, not made their childbearing decisions by the time they are in their late 20's and 30's. These *couples often are in conflict regarding becoming parents.* Facing their *ambivalence* about becoming parents will help them to live comfortably with whatever decision they ultimately make. Third, *couples view the parenthood conflict as if it were primarily the decision to have a baby rather than the decision to parent.*

Fourth, they erroneously think that *something is wrong with them* because they are taking time to make the decision. Fifth, the couple's *style of making their decision will have implications for future family relationships.* That is, the degree to which children are clearly chosen by both spouses and the reasons for having each child will have significance within the family relationship. The couple's understanding of their motives and the process by which they plan their family is essential in their working through their conflicts about parenthood.

Most couples came to either a 6- or 12-hour workshop, the former held on a weekend and the latter held over eight evening sessions. Some couples came for short-term counseling that lasted from 1 to 20 sessions. The 50 couples ranged in age from 25 to 44; the median age was 30 for the women and 32 for the men. Approximately three-fourths of the couples were married; the remainder lived together. A small minority had already decided to have a child and were interested in learning about specifics of childbirth or childrearing. Others wanted help in deciding whether and when to become pregnant. Some wanted information about adoption. The following cases were chosen to illustrate the themes and issues that emerged during the workshops and counseling sessions.

CASE 1

Andy, age 36, has a doctoral degree in biochemistry and recently left an academic position, of his own accord, to start a consulting firm. Anne, age 35, was a preschool teacher who moved into freelance writing and consulting. They had been married 5 years and seemed committed to their marriage. She is the oldest of three and he a middle child of three.

They came to the workshop veering toward never having children; both felt parenthood was not crucial for personal fulfillment. Anne, however, was concerned that she might wake up one morning at age 55 or 60 and feel deep regret that she was "so self-centered." She did not feel parental pressure to bear children. Her parents were deceased. Andy's parents had become grandparents by their other children.

They talked about nonparenthood during the first year they dated, but neither took the discussions very seriously. Anne's work as a teacher of young children influenced her thinking that it is easy "to make a mess of parenting." She felt torn between possible future regret if they did not have a child and more immediate regret if they did become pregnant without clearing up their ambivalence. Because of her age she felt time running out and impelled to decide quickly.

Andy felt financially secure for the first time in his life and was frightened that children would shake his financial stability. His worries included the rising cost of college, housing, and "the millions of things kids need." He dreaded the possibility of working long hours to support his family "just like my dad. I never saw him." He joked about moving beyond biology and waiting until he and Anne were well established in their 40's or 50's. By that time they might work fewer hours, spend more time together, have enough money to hire help for the housework, and have time to enjoy a child. Anne also liked this fantasy. Neither considered adoption or caring for children later in life as an alternative.

In the workshops Anne and Andy considered the following: What would they miss by not having their own child? What would a child add to their lives that they want and do not have now? Has amniocentesis really made it safe for Anne to wait until she is 40 to become pregnant?

Six months after the last workshop session, they reported that, they decided to wait at least a year before making their final decision, to read as much as possible about pregnancy after 35, to save as much money as they could during the year, and to talk to couples who had their children after their mid-30's. Andy researched the economics of having children and discovered that his financial estimations had been inflated. Both reported feeling in better positions to make the decision after having gathered this information. After the year they remained nonparents.

The issues apparent in this first case affect many modern couples. Concerns about earning a good living and anxieties about one's own upbringing influence the decision. Couples seeking professional help are often not aware of the benefits of having children. They can more readily talk about their negative feelings about parenthood than about positive motivations. If ambivalence is a normal stage in the decision-making process, then people also need to see the positive side before making their final decision.

Uncertainties about dealing with one's own and with a child's dependency needs also were manifested. In today's era of "be your own best friend" some worry about sacrificing care of self and spouse for a child. Many of today's couples, raised in families where parenthood was synonomous with self-sacrifice wonder how they might balance the message from the past ("children come first") with the message of the present ("you're entitled to your own life").

Economic inflation, unemployment, and childrearing costs also are threatening to modern couples. Gathering concrete data and information on economic (and medical) factors in childbirth are crucial for adequate decision making.

CASE 2

Another couple came to counseling after talking about having a baby for 4 years "with no resolution in sight." They had reached a state of great conflict and distress and found themselves fighting every time they saw a baby. Bill feared they would soon divorce over the problem; Bunny felt depressed.

They were both 33-year-old lawyers, and worked 12- to 16-hour days. They met during their first year in law school and married the day after graduation. Each was an only child. Bunny felt that they must have two children or none at all. Bill felt less firm about family size, but was intent on becoming a father. He reported feeling "burned out" from working so hard and wanted to slow down. He felt ready to have a child. Bunny was undecided. Bill was angry at her vacillating. She felt that if she had a child at that time, her career would suffer; but if she did not have a child, she risked losing Bill. "What's so good about kids?" she asked "What are you afraid of?" he responded.

They worked in weekly counseling sessions. They imagined how they would feel if Bill worked less and Bunny continued her work schedule. They began to support the idea that they had different needs and expectations about careers and parenthood. Sorting these differences they began evaluating their fused, career-based marriage.

It became clear that they had virtually no experiences as adults with children. It was suggested that they borrow a child. Their experiences with a cousin's 2-year-old were meaningful. Each backed down from the previously rigid stance; Bill saw some of the problems of parenthood, while Bunny saw some of the benefits. They planned to spend more time with children and work less before making a decision. Also, they planned to talk to other dual-career couples, some who worked out sharing child care, and some who chose not to have children. A year later, they reported that they both were working less, had made time for hobbies and friends, including some neighborhood children, and planned to try to become pregnant with the year.

Many contemporary couples have been age-segregated, spending much of their childhood and adulthood with people of their own or near their own ages. For this couple, the failure of our society to prepare people for parenthood was apparent. Feelings that parenthood is mysterious or frightening were reinforced by lack of models for the type of parenting they wanted to create; more sharing between wife and husband of childrearing functions, combining career and parenting for both spouses, and use of nonfamily support services were important to explore.

The birth order of Bunny and Bill was a significant factor. She, an only child, did not want to have only one child; he, one of several, was not so affected.

Concerns and fears on how a child would affect their marriage added to the childbearing decision. Some husbands express fear that they will be excluded from the intimacy of the mother–infant bond, and wonder if they will still be loved as much by their wives. Other spouses, like Bunny, fear dissolution of their marriage if a joint decision cannot be made. Still others, seeing marriages failing, wonder if theirs can withstand the stress of children.

CASE 3

This couple, in their mid-20's had been married for 2 years. Carol, an accountant, recently left her job when the firm she worked for moved to another city. Chuck worked with his father and brothers in the family laundry business. They were both the youngest in families of four children. Discussions at home resulted in Chuck saying that the decision was ultimately Carol's and that he would be happy either way. Carol accused him of backing out and asked him to come for the workshop sessions.

Carol and Chuck grew up in a small, ethnic neighborhood in which most women were mothers by the age of 22. They reported that both sets of parents repeatedly asked when they would "settle down" and start a family. Carol felt that they were beginning to be seen as deviant by their parents and by others. Both talked about not wanting to reject their parents and siblings, but needing to decide on a way of life that was their own.

Carol wanted children. She wanted to see her body change during pregnancy and to have the experience of mothering. Chuck, having one infertile brother was somewhat concerned about his own fertility. Also, he did not feel ready to become a father.

Carol talked about wanting to stay home the first few years of her child's life, but at the same time she questioned the traditional lives of her older siblings and her parents. Her mother's doting on her father angered her. She was proud that Chuck did at least half the cooking. She had recently left a full-time job and was almost obsessed with trying to decide whether to look for another job or to get pregnant. She wanted Chuck to actively participate in the pregnancy decision. She felt alone and angry.

When faced with the suggestion that she might work part-time and mother a child as well, Carol voiced her fears of being home with a baby. She explored her fantasies about motherhood. After several sessions, Chuck found, from a lab test, that he was fertile. He then began to consider parenthood for himself. They examined their relationship to their families and speculated on the impact that being the youngest children had on their feelings of dependency and fears of striking out on their own.

In the last session, they explored issues of sharing childrearing with outsiders so both might continue working. They prac-

ticed asserting views that would differ from those of their
parents. They decided to wait to have a child. Carol found a new
job. After a year, they decided to become pregnant. Carol felt less
dependent upon Chuck's feelings. He wanted to become a father.
She arranged for a part-time position with her new firm. Still
actively individuating from the own families, they originally
were headed toward parenthood via the push of potential grandparents. Finding their own clear road to parenthood took much
strength.

Fertility fears, and the need for separation and individuation from one's parents were apparent for this couple. The effect
of traditional parenting values on perceptions of parenthood
also were evident. Further, the need to consult both members
of a couple, even when one is willing to accept the other's
desires, is clear. Like other couples, they needed to articulate
to each other their hopes and fears.

ADDITIONAL THOUGHTS FOR THERAPISTS OR COUNSELORS

Couples often are divided on the question of having a
child. Sometimes one spouse will take on the role of the pro-
child speaker and the other will oppose having children. These
roles frequently hide the fact that both are ambivalent about
parenthood. When a therapist works with both spouses at the
same time, the possibility that these roles will become rigid or
that the therapy will further divide them is minimized. Working with only one spouse has the potential for increasing the
conflict without providing a setting for its resolution. When
parenting is the question, therapists must be able and willing to
work with the pair.

The therapist begins by examining (1) how long the couple
has been talking about having children; (2) what changes in
feelings and attitudes have occurred over the course of their
relationship; (3) who else has been involved or consulted, what

has been said, and what have been the outcomes of these consultations; and (4) the extent of distress and pressure each person is experiencing. Also, and most important, the therapist will want to assess whether or not the distress stems from underlying marital difficulties. Although most couples benefit from short-term open communication training, some couples require more long-term treatment if their marriage is to survive or if they are to avoid shifting their conflict from one family life-cycle decision to another.

Professionals need to be aware of what questions the couple is openly discussing and what questions are either consciously or unconsciously avoided. Some couples come to therapy wondering if they can resolve their disagreements and remain together as a couple. Most come asking "should we have a baby?" They rarely ask "Do we want to become parents?" Switching the emphasis from having to becoming is an important step in the counseling process.

Couples often are not aware of the rewards of parenting. Some see parents as all-giving and children as all-taking. A therapist must assess the degree of satisfaction each partner feels with the marital relationship and the extent to which each feels fulfillment in other areas of life. Some people come to therapy hoping that, if they have a child, they will somehow be propelled into a new era when they will be "all grown up." Both the fear that they are not yet perfect and the wish that children will transform them should be pointed out.

A therapist also can help couples put parenthood into a longer time perspective. People vary in their ability to imagine different stages of parenthood. Fantasizing the endings to imaginary situations at different stages of parenthood has been valuable in helping people gain a sense that parenthood has a developmental flow. Conveying the notion that parenthood potentially involves change and growth in parents, as well as in children, is helpful for those feeling the pressure of perfectionism.

Some people, in the midst of working out their life priorities, find making commitments difficult. Coming to grips with the fact that any commitment closes the doors to others is a task for people at this transition. Others are working on achieving a sense of what is and what is not under their control. Some couples feel less vulnerable knowing that certain aspects of childbirth and childrearing are theirs to decide. For example, they can choose a method of childbirth or who will deliver their baby. Sorting out inherited, family or cultural myths surrounding children often helps couples to balance the conscious and less conscious aspects of their decision. This process engenders a greater feeling of being in control. Facing the things they cannot control, such as families' reactions to their decisions, the sex of their child, or the temperament of the baby also helps.

Work on spouses' families of origin is important. This might include examining one's birth order position or role in one's family system and the impact of these on feelings about parenthood. Exploring what might have been happening in one's family at the time one was born, how parents were experiencing their lives, and how one's birth was felt in the family can be insightful. Considering feelings about siblings, and their arrival into the family, as well as current feelings and relationships with siblings, is essential.

Therapists may want to help couples focus on the degree of their involvement with families other than their families of origin. Those who work with children in hospitals, schools, or in treatment often are suffering from overexposure to the stresses of parenthood and from a lack of experience with normal and healthy families. Evaluating the degree of isolation lays the groundwork for deciding which suggestions, if any, to make for couples to broaden their contacts with other people.

Last, the therapist works on his or her attitudes toward and experiences in parenting. If the therapist has already made childbearing decisions, examining these and understanding how they were made is crucial if one is to avoid projecting onto others.

Couples or individuals may be looking to professionals for direction, or for the "expert's" answer. Exploring the treatment relationship, the expectations of the couple, and the agenda of the therapist is necessary to dispel unrealistic attitudes towards the therapist and the work.

It is likely that increasing numbers of couples will come for professional advice regarding childbearing decisions. It behooves those of us undertaking this endeavor, whether it be through workshops, therepy, or casual comments to appreciate the complexities surrounding the decision to become parents.

REFERENCES

Bernard, J. *The future of motherhood.* New York: Penguin Books, 1974.

Boston Women's Health Book Collective. *Ourselves and our children.* New York: Random House, 1978.

Boynton, G. M. The relationship between identity development and attitudes toward motherhood in young married professional women. Unpublished doctoral dissertation, Teachers College, Columbia University, 1978.

Cizmar, P. L. Aunt Mary said there'd be days like this: reflections on whether to have a child. *Mother Jones,* 1979, *4*(8), 21–30.

Dreifus, C. Do I want a baby? *McCalls,* 1977, *105*(2), 203ff.

Lederer, W. J., & Jackson, D. D. *The mirages of marriage.* New York: Norton, 1968.

McCauley, C. S. *Pregnancy after 35.* New York: Dutton, 1976.

Nortman, D. Parental age as a factor in pregnancy outcome and child development. *Reports of population/family planning,* No. 16, New York: Population Council, 1974.

Ory, G. The decision to parent or not: Normative and structural components. *Journal of Marriage and the Family,* 1978, *40,* 531–539.

Peck, E. *The baby trap.* New York: Bernard Geis, 1971.

Pohlman, E., Pohlman, J. M. *The psychology of birth planning.* Cambridge, Ma.: Schenkman, 1969.

Radl, S. *Mother's day is over.* New York: Norton, 1973.

Ravich, R. Family adjustment to pregnancy and childbirth. Paper delivered at a conference on The Birth of an American Child, sponsored by the National Institute for the Psychotherapies. New York, N.Y. May 6, 1978.

Veevers, J. E. Voluntarily childless wives: An exploratory study. *Sociology and Social Research,* 1973, *57,* 356–366.

Veevers, J. E. The moral careers of voluntarily childless wives: Notes on the defense of a variant world view. *The Family Coordinator,* 1975, *24,* 473–487.

Whelan, E. M. *A baby? ... maybe.* New York: Bobbs-Merrill, 1975.

Part II

PSYCHOLOGICAL RESPONSES TO PREGNANCY

Pregnancy is a time of heightened psychological sensitivity and responsiveness. Ambivalent emotions and intrapsychic conflicts often manifest themselves in physical symptoms as well as in vivid dreams and fantasies. Some of the psychological responses of expectant parents reflect cultural expectations, others stem from hormonal changes, and still others have their roots in the unique psychological make-up of the individuals involved. The contributors to this section discuss the responses of pregnant women, expectant fathers, and the people with whom they have emotional ties. Many of the papers note that the experience of pregnancy really involves the psychological relationships linking three generations: the unborn child, the prospective parents, and their own mothers and fathers. All of the contributors suggest the enormous importance of a dependable supportive environment for persons experiencing the developmental crisis of pregnancy.

chapter 8

PSYCHOLOGICAL CRISES IN NORMAL PREGNANCY

Patsy Turrini

This chapter discusses psychological experience during normal pregnancies, an area sorely in need of attention and study. The ideas are based primarily upon the work of psychoanalytic theorists (e.g. Benedick, 1973; Bibring, 1959; Deutsch, 1973; Kestenberg, 1978), clinical observations and research conducted at the Mother's Center, Hicksville, New York, research in Developmental Ego Psychology (e.g. Blanck & Blanck, 1974; Hartman, 1958, Jacobsen, 1964, Mahler, 1974) and upon the work of the women's health movement. A brief review of some major contributions of each of these positions to understanding pregnancy will be presented first; a description of psychological experiences during the course of pregnancy and case examples will follow.

Bibring (1959) introduced the concept of pregnancy as a *maturational crisis*. She observed severe psychological disturbances in pregnant women who had no previous history of psychopathology or symptomatology. She concluded, and other theorists have concurred, that pregnancy represents a crisis that is resolved only after the child is born. Further, she noted, that therapeutic intervention provides rather immediate relief of the symptoms.

Research at the Mother's Center focuses on factors affecting mothers' self-esteem, self-representations, and the maternal ego ideal. The studies take place a year or more after the pregnancy. Using an exploratory study vehicle, the Post Natal Questionnaire, the events of the pregnancy are reconstructed. Evidence to date has suggested that there are traumas experienced in normal pregnancy and delivery that are laid down in memory states with affect attached to these memories. The memories reside largely in the unconscious or preconscious. The research also indicates that there are some universal psychic developmental crises in pregnancy as well as unique individual responses.

Psychoanalytic developmental ego psychology, which began with Freud was dramatically augmented by the publication in 1939 (1958 in the United States) of Hartman's "Ego Psychology and the Problem of Adaption." Hartman proposed that the infant *arrives* into the world with a set of inborn ego apparatus of primary automomy, which then interact in the *average expectable environment.* The unfolding of the ego apparatus and the psychoanalytic study of normal development became primary foci of the ego developmentalists.

The women's movement and the women's health movement have challenged and helped in the advancement of our understanding of the developmental and health needs of the female, as well as of the male. *Our bodies Ourselves* (Boston Women's Health Collective, 1975) noting an example of one of the best writings from the movement, has an excellent chapter on childbearing.

Ego psychology and the women's movement have in common the appreciation that people are a product of their birth and interaction with the environment. They also share the belief that a phenomenon of specific behavior should be appreciated for its adaptation to survival. Further, they both would reject labeling and prejudicial views of women's behavior.

Waelder's (1936) concept of the priniciple of multiple function also is relevant to understanding experiences during normal pregnancies. Waelder proposed that a "double or generally multiple conception of each psychic action is altogether necessary in the light of psychoanalysis." The principle of multiple function states that even if a psychic act is an attempted solution for one definite problem, it must also, at the same time and in some way, be an attempted solution for other problems; that is, any psychic act is to be understood as the expression of the collective function of the total organism. Pregnancy serves a multiple of psychic needs, and the specific behavior of a pregnant woman is a result of multiple determinants.

The discussion to follow is limited to crises experienced in normal pregnancies. The focus is on the "good enough mother," a term used by Winnicott (1953), in an uncomplicated pregnancy. The good enough mother is defined herein as the person with a structured ego with self-protective functions. She has the capacity for psychological parenthood; as distinguished from mothers who only have a capacity for biological motherhood. Blum (1978) highlighted this distinction in the concept of *the maternal ego ideal,* a substructure of the ego ideal, which resides in the superego. It is the ideal state of the woman's internalizations of how she would like to be as a mother. The ego ideal contains determined by many sources, but it is mainly organized by her experiences with her own mother and father. It is a crucial substructure within the personality that organizes the act of protective nurturing.

The following discussion considers only five of the hundreds of "crises" that the good enough mother experiences in a normal pregnancy.

THE DECISION TO BECOME PREGNANT

The decision to become pregnant may not be made consciously and the attempt to make this decision may in and of itself cause an intrapsychic or interpsychic crisis. The female,

more often, has the stronger conscious driving force in determining the pregnancy. The male tends to follow the lead. She
is more consciously determined and more in pursuit of a child.
Although the following example is extreme, it highlights this
hypothesis. In one of our postnatal exploratory survey groups,
five out of seven women reported that they "pulled the plug"
(i.e., consciously did not use the diaphragm unbeknownst to
their husbands.) They suffered shame and guilt about their
decisions.

As a result of greater freedom of choice in choosing childbearing, young people are thrown into a confusion of *how* to
decide to become pregnant. What justifies a decision to bring
a child into this world? As one woman said, "I can't just decide
to have a child for my own happiness." She was acknowledging
that having a child would give her pleasure and that this "too
selfish" proposition did not recognize the needs of the "other"
(the child and her husband). We might call this confusion a
normal conflict residing in the intrasystemic conflict within the
ego ideal, and an intersystemic conflict between the id and
superego. To have a child is, in fact, based on the pleasure
principle and the right to pleasure is not so easily attained in
our culture, despite the fact that we tend to see, on the surface,
pleasure-seeking adults. Being able to have pleasure *without
guilt* often is quite difficult for the unanalyzed person.

Unconscious pleasures are obtained and gratified in having
a child. Freud and others postulated on the psychosexual matu-
ration line that the baby is equated with breast-feces-penis, as
well as being longed for as the ultimate gift to and union with
the father.

An active conscious decision to have a child, therefore,
calls up unconscious determinants, sometimes producing guilt
Kohut's (1971) proposed that the gleam in the mother's eye is
a beacon which influences the child's perception of self and
behavior. I have observed clinically that if the parents have
discouraged the child from reproducing (and this does happen),
it has a profound influence on the motive for nonchildbearing.

The grandparents-to-be's wish for a child, a wish determined by their own generativity, has a basic positive influence on the child's freedom to have a child. Having healthy parents who can love themselves encourages the birth of the next generation.

Neugarten's (1972) study of social clocks indicates that we are influenced to adjust to a perceived timetable for life's events. So, for example, we say, we graduated on time; or we married later than most; or we had our baby earlier than some. We judge ourselves against a timetable. She cited the following facts in a paper presented at the American Psychoanalytic Conference: "In 1920, a woman left school at 14, married at 22, had her first child at 24, and her last born child at 42. Her husband died when she was 53, and her last child married when she was 55. She usually was widowed before her last child left home. Today, a woman leaves school at 18, is married at 20, has her first child before 21, and her last child at 26. At 32 her last child is in full-time school, and her last child leaves home when she is 48. Her husband will die when she is 64, and she will live to be 80." Looking at the facts, we can see that a timetable does in fact exist.

Consider another framework. A real family consists of four people. If you are a family of five or three, you are not conforming to the model, and might feel cultural pressure. You are either underpopulating or overpopulating. Our research on the mother of the only child indicated that she suffers extensively from being told she is selfish and obviously raising a spoiled child. One determinant of these remarks stems from the jealousy of those who have had siblings, and have longed for exclusivity with their parents. (Arlow, 1972).

Other people's timetables and views may not have a direct bearing on what we do but the degree to which we are unable to separate or individuate psychologically is the degree to which we may make decisions on others' timetables, or may suffer from considereable criticism if we have differed from the norm.

DOES THIS CHILD EXIST?

Active psychic preparation for parenthood begins with the first missed menstrual period. At this point, however, the only things that are changing in the woman's life are some body features and internal silent physiological processes. Prior to quickening there is enlargement of the breasts, fatigue, some weight gain, and perhaps some morning sickness—body signals that are signs of pregnancy. Few women report any conscious knowledge of the conception or early detection of the fetus. Questions aroused by these body changes include: What is the self and what is the baby? Am I pregnant or not? Should I begin psychological readiness for mothering? Should I announce the pregnancy? There is great fear about announcing a pregnancy and many attitudes color the decision. The superstition exists for some that to think about a healthy baby tempts the hand of fate. This message is frequently taught by the parents, but, also, resides in the harsh superego of the woman herself. The good enough mother frequently suffers from a harsh superego. A critical conflict develops: should she think about being pregnant or not. When the healthy ego, fueled by self-protective functions and ideals of the maternal ego ideal wins, the good enough mother enters into a constant monitoring of her health and of the health of the fetus. On trips to the bathroom, for example, the woman watches for staining, one signal to her of the safety of the fetus. A life and death detection process goes on in the conscious experience, privately, and alone in the bathroom.

The event of quickening brings "great relief." The first physiological response of the baby is often described as a feeling of a bubble or gas. Therefore, the obstetrician's listening with the stethescope for the heartbeat is a most momentous dramatic event. We have recorded a common reporting of the terrible fear a woman feels while she waits, for what seems endless hours, in a deafening silence, for the physician's verdict. Is there a baby? Is the baby alive? Zimmerman et al. (1977) quotes one woman: "Someone told me I should feel life at the end of my third month. When I went for my check-up I could hardly stand up, I was so sure I was carrying a dead baby."

At this stage a woman has a strong dependence on her obstetrician and the obstetrical equipment. Awaiting the verdict from the stethescope reading deepens the woman's perception of the physician as critical to the life and death of her baby. The physician's knowledge of the use of the stethescope intimidates and influences feelings of self-inadequacy that become set in motion in pregnancy. A group in San Francisco have a storefront pregnancy center where the women take their own urine and blood pressure tests, and use the stethescope. At last report, they were planning to integrate a pregnancy check center within the local hospital where the women would use the obstetrical equipment themselves. It seems that the more active, the more knowledgeable, the more self-protective a woman can be early in the pregnancy, the more her feelings of resourcefulness and competence can be set in motion.

Decisions women will make during pregnancy by deciding on a particular doctor and hospital have grave consequences. That decision basically determines the type of prenatal care and delivery she and the child will experience. She may be in a crisis state a day, month, or years later as a result of that decision. Overcoming the memory of the psychoticlike state she was in while under the influence of scopolamine, or bearing the pain or hindsight awareness of having chosen a delivery that caused a learning disability in the child are traumas with lasting effects (Turrini, 1977). Therapeutic help to rework the memories can bring relief, but she will suffer from chronic sorrow.

THE LAST 6 WEEKS OF PREGNANCY

Although the whole of pregnancy has been termed a catastrophe, the last 6 weeks of a pregnancy might be considered a disaster. Here follows a composite image of the state of things, some of which is drawn from the text in *Our Bodies Ourselves* (1975):

> The stomach is pushed up by the uterus and flattened. Indigestion is common. There is shortness of breath and pressure on the lungs from the uterus. The diaphragm may be moved up as much as an inch. There may be difficulty getting a breath. The body is heavy, and walking becomes different in order to effect the proper balance, often leaning back to counteract the heavier front. Backaches occur. Hemmorhoids, constipation, are common, as are varicose veins and stretch marks. The body is in a total state of change. Bending over is impossible, and the protruding abdomen prevents looking at the feet. The Braxton Hicks contractions are frequent, and are quite painful for some women. The baby is very active and kicks may cause bruising and disturb sleep. Activities are sorely restricted. Many women can no longer fit behind the wheel of the car.

Psychic preparation for delivery is complete prior to the last 6 weeks of pregnancy, and the woman is as ready as she ever will be to deliver at the beginning of the last 6 weeks. Completion of psychic preparation for delivery is defined as the acceptance of the reality of the coming baby, an attachment to, yet differentiation and individuation from the longed-for baby. Although there is some controversy on this point, the last 6 weeks do not seem to serve a function in psychic preparation time for delivery. The time hangs heavily. Working women have by this time left their employment, and are beginning to experience isolation, boredom, and the impact from all that it means to be suddenly unemployed. It is the time of the beginning glimmer of the "I felt like I fell off the end of the world" syndrome. In this period resides the looking and listening for the awaited signal for the beginnings of labor. The awareness that there is no way to affect the onset of labor leads to an increase in fears and peculiar thoughts. One woman reported that everytime the phone rang, she thought that she was being called to inform her that labor had begun. Although there are joyful feelings in this period, evidence indicates that there are morbid feelings, not to mention the particularly conflicting feelings about sexual behavior in this period.

We have repeatedly observed that women experience a mild depression if they do not deliver on the due date. The longer the time goes beyond the date, the greater the intensity of the depression. Fears about the babies' health increase rapidly. The delay seems to symbolize an image of a defect, or a "something has gone wrong" sensation.

THE ONSET OF LABOR

The onset of labor creates a crisis. All good childbirth preparation courses aim at reducing these fears. Such instructions as: "When you begin labor, do not panic, do not wake your husband, as he will need his sleep for later" reflect interventions to reduce fear. It is too bad that it does not work. When the first contraction hits, when the bloody mucous discharge is observed, if the water breaks, whatever the signal, the woman is on red-alert. She is internally mobilized to arrange conditions to properly deliver a healthy baby. This event needs more intensive study. Perhaps there is a species-specific, i.e., preprogrammed genetically determined behavior that is set in motion at the onset of labor. Klaus & Kennell (1976) describe it this way:

> Detailed and precise observations of many species have shown that adaptive species-specific patterns of behaviour—including *nesting*, exploring, grooming and retrieving—before, during and after parturition, have evolved to meet the needs of the young in the animal's usual environment. For example, the domestic cat, whether in Russia, the United States, or England, behaves in a characteristic way at the time of the birth of her kittens.

If, as I believe, a species-specific behavior exists, it works in combination with the healthy developed ego functions. A mother is capable of mothering as a result of a combination of these structures and forces. Consider then, that the signs in early labor stimulate instinctual "nesting" activity. What starts to go wrong is that others are not in tune with the woman's feelings in early labor. Our culture has arranged for her to be alone during the beginning of labor. Research has indicated that women do a fine job of going through the early labor process alone, putting aside their needs and fears and mounting terror about the delivery. As one woman described, "When labor began I went out to get food. I was standing in line at McDonald's buying food for the other children, when it hit me, 'This is a funny place to be.' " She suddenly became aware of her aloneness, and the inappropriate place for a delivery.

In our studies, women report feelings of extreme fright during early labor. Any time in life that one experiences strong feelings of fright or helplessness, a resulting scar image will be laid down. Therefore, psychological scars result from fears of labor.

A particular phenomenon observed repeatedly that creates more of a crisis in early labor is the assumption of certain "indisputable truisms" of the medical team. An article in the living section of *Newsday,* March 13, 1978 entitled: "Bouquets for Unlikely Midwives" reflected this phenomenon:

> Mrs. Pope, age 31, was not due to deliver for another two weeks ... but she began having labor pains while lying on the couch. "My father," said Mrs. Pope, "called the fire department, and they were in contact with our Doctor. He (the doctor) said it must be false labor pains. But the fire chief said, 'No way. She's giving birth right now.' They (the firemen) did all the work. The baby came out and they wrapped him up and clamped up the umbilical cord.' " The truth is that no one can predict the course of the labor nor the timing of the delivery. (p.7)

Women are repeatedly told that they should enter the hospital when they have 3-minute regular contractions. The majority of women in our studies indicated there is "no such thing as a regular 3-minute contraction." A commonly reported pattern in early labor is a 10-minute, 3-minute, 12-minute, 5-minute, 10-minute contraction pattern. Women accept the myth of the regular 3-minute contraction, and become additionally confused and frightened about where to be during early labor. Furthermore, they assume that their irregularity is peculiar to them and representative of their being abnormal. We have had reports from women of being rejected from entry into the hospital because of irregular contractions. In one reported incident, the family went home, the mother tried to keep calm during increasingly intense contractions, and when she could stand it no longer, they rushed back to the hospital. Then she was required to go through the admission procedure and then placed on the stretcher in the hall. When she said she was about to deliver, the physician told her not to push. Two minutes later she delivered the child, alone in the hospital hallway. The physician screamed that she could have killed the baby and ripped her insides out by having pushed. This same woman reported having difficulty in bonding in the early period with her baby. The inhumane care she received and the accusation made, I interpret, caused her to feel a terrible sense of inadequacy. The truth is that there are irregular contractions, and that the 3-minute contraction is not an appropriate signal for entering the hospital.

The simple solution for humane care in early labor is that a woman should be with an empathic aware person who is knowledgable and able to help her deliver. Being alone is an excessive strain. Having someone to ask questions of, and being in a place where the woman knows she can deliver comfortably, is essential to her mental health in early labor. Early labor lounges, where families can be together and move about would be better for the mental health of the husband, too.

LABOR AND OBSTRETRICAL INTERVENTION

The effects of obstetric tools, e.g., fetal monilers, forceps, the strapped labor table, the intravenous bottle on women's behavior also must be considered. Feridian's introduction to Lang's (1972) *The Birth Book* traces the history of forceps in obstetrical care.

> In 1598, the Chamberlain brothers invented the forceps, but kept them selfishly as a family secret until the latter half of the 17th Century. The forceps were of extreme value in certain deliveries, but unfortunately, when the use of this tool became popularized, it began to be used needlessly in uncomplicated cases without warrant. With the introduction of such skilled manipulations, men once again entered the profession of midwifery. It is of great significance that the attendance of male midwives followed closely upon the introduction of forceps into childbirth. In the late 1600's, Mauriceau first began to deliver his childbearing "Patients" in bed. In America, Dewees introduced the back delivery in the mid 1800's. Previously, and dating to antiquity, women had given birth squatting, seated on the obstetrical stool, or upon the lap of another woman. With Mauriceau's intervention, the woman was placed flat on her back, a position which offers a fine view to the performing physician, but is in total defiance to the active forces of gravity. Nor does this position encourage the laboring woman to utilize her own efforts in delivery.

Obstetrical teams do not exactly have a perfect track record in the use of equipment, yet many persons are in awe of machinery. Roberto Caldero-Barcia, past-President of the International Federation of Gynecologists and Obstetricians, and director of the Latin American Center for Perinatology and Human Development of the World Health Organization has described (1975) the extreme deleterious effects to the baby of the early breaking of the amniotic sac to stimulate labor, thereby removing the protective cushion for the baby's head as it moves and bangs down the birth canal. Mehl (1976) has reported the damage to the infant's head through the use of forceps. These are but two of the frightening results of the use of obstetrical equipment during birth.

Research continues to suggest that certain birth practices may have consequences to the fetus which can cause severe organic difficulties, minimal brain dysfunction, and even death. It is the work of a few people, like Doris Haire (e.g. 1972), which has brought to public awareness, and which has begun to raise the consciousness of the community to the cataclysmic effects that can occur through the use of obstetrical equipment.

The challenge in regard to the use of obstetrical equipment is that all parties involved in pregnancy and delivery must be aware of the ramifications of its use, both psychologically and physiologically, both to the mother and to the child. The physician alone should not make all the decisions. The parents should have the opportunity to have full knowledge of the type of equipment that may be used, alternative approaches, and then be in the position to participate actively with the obstetrical team in the decision-making process. It is essential that medical and nonmedical people work together to assure the most optimal delivery possible.

Issues fop the Therapist or Counselor

Critical to helping women in pregnancy is a proper diagnostic assessment. It must be appreciated that certain psychic developmental tasks of pregnancy are universal to all pregnant women. The major body changes in a short period of time and the challenge of attaching to, yet differentiation out from the developing baby are two of the critical tasks. It must be recognized that the women with well-developed ego functions (the good enough mother) will be deeply challenged by these tasks. Some denial, regression in the service of the ego, and mood states of depression, anxiety, unusual fears, and guilt can be considered normal in pregnancy. Women with less structured egos, and less self-protective functions, particularly those without object constancy, will experience severe stress and will need even greater support and help.

It must be recognized in diagnostic assessment that external events will have a potentially damaging effect on the pregnant women's mental health, and therapists need to know what these are, and help women anticipate what will be of help to them, what will facilitate their growth, so that scars can be prevented. We must find ways to use the maturational crisis of pregnancy, the obstetrical tools, the setting in which she gives birth to promote growth, maturity, confidence, a positive body image, and a sense of well-being. Women should be encouraged to be active, to learn more about their bodies and its capacity and strength to overcome previously inhibiting fears, and to rise to their optimal capacities. Therapists must come to appreciate the cataclysmic effects of pregnancy and parenting and to have full knowledge of this subject.

CONCLUSION

The traumas associated with pregnancy are laid down in memory states residing largely in the unconscious and affect is attached to these memories. When a woman says everything was fine for her, she consciously believes that. The repressed memories, however, can drain energies away from more positive self-esteem within herself, and away from the interchange in bonding with her child. The Post Natal Questionnaire used at the Mother's Center is one tool which enables women to work through the pregnancy and birth trauma (Turrini, 1977). Not only does the Mothers' Center help women get relief with this hindsight experience, it is a gathering place to complement programs which will prevent trauma to the mother, father, and child.

It is hoped that the psychiatric, social work, psychological, and nursing communities will attend to the critical psychic components affecting members of the family in pregnancy and childbirth. These psychic phenomena must be researched, catalogued, and the findings disseminated. Can anyone dispute the fact that healthy children born into a healthy family is the basis for a sound sane society?

REFERENCES

Arlow, J. The only child. *Psychoanalytic quarterly,* 1972 *61* (4,) 507–536.

Benedek, T. Psychological aspects of mothering. Parenting as a developmental phase, *Psychoanalytic investigations.* New York: Quandrangle/The New York Times, 1973.

Bibring, G. Some considerations of the psychological process in pregnancy, *The Psychoanalytic study of the child, 14:* 113–121.

Blanck, G., & Blanck, R. *Ego psychology: Theory and practice,* New York: Columbia University Press, 1974.

Blum, H. The maternal ego ideal, Unpublished paper. New York, March, 1978.

Boston Womens Health Collective. *Our bodies ourselves.* Boston: Simon & Schuster, 1975.

Caldeyro-Barcia, R. Obstetric intervention: It's effect on the fetus and newborn Part II. Paper presented at the *Obstetrical Management and Infant Outcome: Implications for Future Mental and Physical Development.* Wednesday, April 9, 1975, New York.

Deutsch, H. *The Psychology of Women, Volume II: Motherhood,* New York: Bantam Books, 1973.

Freud, S. (1909) Analysis of a phobia in a five-year old boy. *The Collected works of Sigmund Freud* Vol. 10, London: Hogarth Press, 1955.

Haire, D. *The cultural warping of childbirth.* Seattle: International Childbirth Education Association, 1972.

Hartman, H. *Ego psychology and the problem of adaptation.* New York: International Universities Press, 1958.

Bouquets for unlikely midwives. *Newsday,* March 13, 1978.

Jacobson, E. *The self and the object world.* New York: International Universities Press, 1964.

Kestenberg, J. Regression and reintegration in pregnancy. *Journal of the American Psychoanalytic Association,* 1976, *24,* 243–250.

Klaus, M. & Kennell, J. *Maternal and infant bonding.* St. Louis. Mosby, 1976.

Kohut, H. *The analysis of the self.* New York: International Universities press, 1971.

Lang, R. Introduction. *The birth book.* Palo Alto, Cal: Genesis Press, 1972.

Mahler, M. Pine, F. Bergman, A. *The Psychological Birth of the Human Infant,* Basic Books, Inc., 1975.

Mehl, L. Statistical outcome of home births in the U.S., current status *Safe alternatives in childbirth.* Chapel Hill, N.C.: National Association of Parents and Professionals for Safe Alternatives in Childbirth, (NAPSAC), 1976.

Neugarten, B. Social Clocks, A paper presented at the American Psychoanalytic Association. New York, December, 1972.

Turrini, P. A Mothers Center: Research, Service and Advocacy. *Social Work Journal.* 1977, *22,* (6), 478–483.

Waelder, R. The principle of multiple function. *The psychoanalytic quarterly,* 1936, *5,*

Winnicott, D. W. "Transitional objects and transitional phenomena, *International Journal of Psychoanalysis,* 1953, *34.*

Zimmerman, H. Turrini, P. Weiss, S. Slepian, L. A mothers center, women work for social change. *Children Today,* 1977, 11–13. *6,* (2).

chapter 9

PSYCHOLOGICAL AND PHYSICAL WARNING SIGNALS REGARDING PREGNANCY
Early Psychotherapeutic Intervention

Joan Offerman-Zuckerberg

We are all used to hearing of the notion of "warning signals" regarding physical illness. For example, in cancer there are certain bodily evidences that we become alert to: sores that do not heal, or an unusual lump. We are used to hearing of the notion of warning signals regarding heart disease: pains in the chest and changes in blood pressure that may be alarming. We become careful about diet, life stress, and exercise, running miles daily in an effort to counterbalance the body's accumulation of disease and inadequate care. If we have fever, we think illness, and we may measure it with a thermometer and take appropriate medication. Such judicial steps, however, taken so naturally for physical disorders are not taken so naturally when we find ourselves in the context of a psychological condition. Pregnancy is a psychological and physical condition, involving for the person a major developmental step. It is accompanied by psychological upheaval, and can precipitate change in our sense of self and our relationship to significant others. It can test our capacity for intimacy and attachment, over time and into the future.

Undoubtedly, we could be better educated regarding the possible "warning signals" of pregnancy maladaption. Some warning signals are purely psychological in nature, and may include: (1) excessive worries and/or fears regarding damage to self during pregnancy, damage to the future child, to the marriage, or to the parents; (2) unusual fantasies or thoughts, experienced as "out of control"; (3) acute and prolonged separation anxiety; (4) loss of emotional responsiveness; (5) unusual mood swings; and (6) resistance to "nestbuilding" behavior. The signals may be more physical in nature and may include: (1) habitual abortion; (2) hypertension; (3) undue nausea; (4) inappropriate weight gain; (5) unusual and vague aches, cramps, and pains in the genital area; (6) blushing, flushing, and fainting; (7) breathing difficulties; (8) gastrointestinal complaints; and (9) circulation problems and general aches and pains. These symptoms exist along a continuum of severity from normal, i.e., occuring in a majority of women, to abnormal. By sensitizing ourselves to the signals and to the possibility of their underlying meanings, we are attending to something that may lead to effective, therapeutic prevention of possible psychological disturbance, for the mother, father, and future child.

This psychological and physical focus relates to a holistic understanding of the person and one that, if applied, can facilitate into action the model of early "primary prevention." The concept of warning signals leads to the notion of a self-administered "psychological check-up"[1] given at a time when motivation for health is at a peak. As a result, a woman might consider visiting a psychologist in much the same way as one might go to the obstetrician when pregnant, for a check-up, perhaps, in each trimester of the pregnancy and several visits postpartum. The visit may be prompted not only because of pathology or the

---

[1] The concept of a "psychological checkup" came out of a discussion with a colleague, Henry Seiden.

presence of alarming warning signals, but because pregnancy is being regarded as an important psychological and physical event. If there are certain stresses, questions, or confusions, it would be appropriate to speak to someone adequately informed and responsive. The model proposed, and it remains in the working stage, is obstetrician/midwives working with psychiatrists, psychologists, social workers, and other trained mental health professionals, during pregnancy, and the first year postpartum.

It is perhaps curious to discover that how pregnancy is perceived and assimilated by the expectant mother, her feelings attending this perception, and the attitudes and motivations involved are areas that psychology has relatively neglected. It is curious in that pregnancy and childbirth are natural phenomena involving complex psychological states occurring in the majority of women. Many investigators regard pregnancy as "the initial home for the child," in both a psychological and biological sense. Pregnancy may, moreover, be viewed as a psychological and physical preparation for maternal functioning, marking the beginning of a mother's relationship to her child and between the husband and wife as parents (Tanzer, 1967). Finally, from any theoretical perspective, pregnancy and childbirth can be understood as an important developmental crisis in a woman's life, one involving adaptation as well as profound physiological change. Some writers compare it to adolescence in terms of the degree of psychological upheaval and of emotional lability. Indeed, Rorschach Inkblot Tests results of pregnant women are comparable to those of adolescents in the incidence of fluid, transitional signs relating to emotional lability, psychic upheaval, and imminent, reactive worries and concerns. The pregnant woman is ordinarily quite willing and motivated to be open. Pregnant women's responses to the Pregnancy Thematic Apperception Test (PTAT) (Knobel, 1967; Zuckerberg, 1972) are rich in elaboration, with a high level of both responsiveness and receptivity to the original stimulus. This responsiveness and concomitant motivation suggests the possibility of a rapidly occurring and positive working alliance between the pregnant woman and the professional. The drive, positive motivation, and feelings of confidence in women with planned pregnancies adds power, moreover, to possible therapeutic bonds.

Three additional factors have provided the impetus for the consideration of psychological consultation for pregnant women with emphasis on psychosomatic warning signals. The understanding of the psychosomatic aspects of pregnancy has as its ultimate research aim the prevention of possible abnormalities of mother and child. Second, the approach may help in the understanding and prevention of the high incidence of postpartum depression, which causes psychological harm to the child, the mother, and the family, and a high incidence of early bonding disturbances in the mother–child interaction. The third impetus comes from personal experience. While I was in the hospital to deliver my second child, a "natural" group formed among the women in the ward. It was dramatic to observe a powerful need among the women to talk. They spoke of both depression and elation, and of a uniform sense of loss and gain as it relates to the baby's "symbiotic rupture" from the body and the beginning process of attachment. We all shared notes, watching eagerly for cues of response and recognition from the child. This experience reinforced the notion that there is a unique readiness to share this event and willingness usually to accept help.

THEORETICAL CONTRIBUTIONS

Many authors regard pregnancy as a "transitional crisis," a time in which psychological defenses are loosened, and a time in which unconscious material is apt to emerge. This emergence can be viewed as being adaptive as it represents an effort to resolve primary conflicts with the woman's mother. Also common to these theories is the crucial significance attributed to the role of fantasy and its influence on physical well-being. There is a significant increase in fantasy activity in pregnant women. For example, as a therapist, it was a challenge to go through two pregnancies and conduct psychotherapy. It took more work and energy to be engaged with the other, as the pressure is to withdraw more, to gaze inward, and to have fantasies and waking dreams. This inward pressure needs to be listened to and perhaps cherished, for it provides the rich soil for fantasy-preparation and narcissistic refueling, a vital part of pregnancy adaptation. Therefore, it can feel stressful to relate to another person intensely, given the counterpressure to let go to a natural and needed refueling process. Also emphasized in these theories is the general increase in primary narcisscism, i.e., the increased attention to self. This is accompanied by the preparation of vast expenditures of energy needed for maternal functioning. Nest-building does not occur after birth, it occurs during pregnancy —in action, as well as in fantasy, feeling, and thought. One starts preparing the child's room and accumulating supplies for the child during pregnancy. This, all in the service of preparation for the child, represents normal preparation for welcoming a separate human being into one's life. There are fantasies about what he or she is going to be like, and there is name giving, both instances of psychological nestbuilding. In groups, women talk about cleaning the oven repetitively, or washing dishes more than usual, or cleaning out drawers. Sometimes a husband will humorously mention "she's never been so neat." Again, this may be viewed as psychological nestbuilding. Psychoanalytically oriented theorists agree that pregnancy involves shifts in the level of distribution of narcissistic libido and object libido, with an increase in narcissism, so that there might be complaints from the husband that there is not enough attention being paid to him. He may become depressed, particularly after quickening, because the pregnant woman now experiences a reality that she did not before. There is now a "real" child and further fantasies of the child to come are evoked.

The psychological steps during pregnancy fundamentally

include incorporation and differentiation. The mother must accept and incorporate the fetus. Some women have trouble with incorporation and some of the signs of this trouble might be translated into physical and/or psychological symptoms, such as undue nausea, habitual abortion, unusual degree of complaining, rumination, and obsessional thinking. Many women have problems with the fact that there is something growing inside the body that is going on despite their conscious effort and control. For some women, who have a particular need "to be in control," this might pose a conflict. Incorporation is the first psychological task that a woman has to master in being pregnant. After quickening, the fetus must be recognized as an object, i.e., a future child, rather than as a part of the self. This involves working through the separation and individuation phases within the woman's own life and then as it applies to the child. Attachment and separation are critical issues that go on constantly in pregnancy, after birth, and, throughout the life cycle. This process is in the service of adaptation, preparing the woman for the eventual separation that goes on after birth. Conflicts regarding this separation can usually be viewed as precipitating problems in postpartum adjustment. The final task of childbearing is birth and acceptance of the loss from the body. The separation is sometimes felt as immense and it can be accompanied by normal feelings of depression.

Underlying the psychological work specific to the pregnancy state, is the ongoing flux of material related to maternal identification and identity. The pregnant woman is renegotiating the developmental issues related to separateness, autonomy, and dependency from her mother. She is working through once again oedipal themes centering on competition, guilt, and retaliation. In the act of pregnancy, the woman is becoming a mother, and, in that way, she is stepping into her mother's shoes and competing with her. It is with this renegotiation that a high incidence of dreams, sleeping, and waking may be activated, and it is with this work that major developmental strides may be taken. The transition to motherhood involves clarification of one's sense of self in a nurturant caretaker role, in a relationship to one's husband as partner, in a relationship to a dependent child, and in a relationship to one's parents. These clarifications, once accomplished, can be accompanied by feelings of self-worth and esteem. If not accomplished, or left unresolved, the psychological system may signal alarm.

Psychosomatic Theory

Psychosomatic theory, as well, underlies the notion of physical warning signals of pregnancy adaptation. The uterus, a muscle, reacts like any other set of muscles in the body to emotional states. Thus, it contracts in states of anger, fear, arousal or sexual excitement. Somatic symptoms during pregnancy may represent repressed feelings or affect concomitants which result from the daming up of emotional expression. They may express directly an emotional state, such as helplessness, or they may indicate ego deficiencies in a person who is unable to resort to fantasy, or intellectual means of controlling anxiety. The role of stress and the individual's constitutionally predetermined response to it, is also an influential factor, which can be conceptualized as "somatic response style." If a woman is apt to somaticize prior to pregnancy; if understress, she has headaches, or symptomatizes in the form of an ulcer or skin rash (whatever the particular pattern of conditioning is) chances are there will be some "somaticization" under stress during pregnancy. It is plausible that a combination of factors operate on some level of simultaneous occurrence, so that there exists a "psychophysical parallelism" with respect to thought, feeling, and body. The question of which comes first—the body symptom or the worry—is, at best, misleading. It is happening in a parallelism, as do most psychological and physical events. Any thought, feeling or impulse we have can very naturally be charged with such emotion that our physical system reacts in simultaneous fashion.

Wittkower et al. (1969) summarizes the psychoanalytic models of the possible relationship between psyche and soma: (1) psychosomatic symptoms may be symbolically meaningful, with the specific symptom symbolizing a repressed feeling; (2) psychosomatic symptoms having no specific meaning but result from the daming up of emotional expression; and (3) psychosomatic symptoms which result from general ego deficits in the ability to use fantasy and verbal mediation to integrate conflicts in the psychic sphere.

It is important to note that excessive somatization is a "regressive" phenomenon and points to ego weakness, poor emotional controls, and usually characterological immaturity. This complex of factors together with a highly charged, ambivalent content, i.e., perhaps a conflicted pregnancy, can signal alarm to the system. Additional stress comes from a rather dependent, ambivalent relationship to one's mother. A warning signal then can come from a multiple based source, physiological vulnerability, psychological predisposition toward somatization, characterological immaturity, and a highly charged psychological situation.

EMPIRICAL STUDIES

Experimental research has pointed to hyperemesis gravidarum (undue nausea), habitual abortion, infertility, toxemia (hypertension), and pseudocyesis (false pregnancy) as the five core psychosomatic conditions, the gross warning signals of a maladaptive pregnancy. Problems in conception and then difficulty holding one's baby may be physical in nature but the research seems to indicate the presence of relevant psychological issues. The above physical states have been associated with conflicts regarding one's relationship to one's mother, and rejection of the female role. Researchers have talked about a cluster of the symptoms as being associated with characterological immaturity, i.e., the woman who is not ready to be a mother and/or who has undue dependency ties on her own mother. If there is residual immaturity, dependency, or hostility toward the mother, the pregnant woman may have a high incidence of psychosomatic complaints manifested as "warning signals." If a problematic relationship to one's mother is not counterbalanced sufficiently by growth-promoting forces present in the woman's life situation and marriage, then this problematic identification with the mother will have a greater likelihood of evidencing itself in psychosomatic warning signals. These problems also may be displaced unconsciously onto the obstetrician/midwife, the woman's body, the husband and marriage, or the self, and may take the form of psychological warning signals. Further displacement onto the woman's mother, father, or finally onto the future child may occur. This displacement may mark the beginning of a family neurosis. One of the reasons, then, for intervention during pregnancy is to monitor more carefully this projective-displacing process.

An illustration of a "psychosomatic" sign and the therapeutic effects of "bonding" are found in the case of an 18-year-old amenorrheic woman referred for suicidal depression. One of the first results of treatment (after four sessions) was the oncoming of menstruation, which, in this case, was related to forming, perhaps for the first time, an unambivalent, positive bond with a woman, the female therapist. This highly charged emotional bond can be said to initiate a series of hormonal changes. Additional factors related to female dysfunction are excessive fears concerning pregnancy, childbirth, and motherhood. Fears during pregnancy can include feelings of bodily distortion, a general sense of damage to the body, and the fear of losing control. There may be, in addition, feelings of being drained by a parasitic fetus. There may be insecurities and inadequacies about becoming a mother for the first time and the competitive oedipal pressure from one's own mother. All of this in excessive degree may lead to somatic symptomatology during pregnancy. Also, there is the general factor of characterological immaturity and dependency on the mother which can outweigh all of these variables.

Heinstein (1967) obtained data from 156 clinic patients and discovered that women who were moody or easily upset, (a subtle psychological warning signal), or who felt dull and indifferent (indifference can mean that emotion is being dammed up) encountered a significant degree of physical complications during pregnancy. Women who have severe depression and withdrawal symptoms experienced significantly more serious complications during the whole course of pregnancy and in delivery as well. There have been consistent correlations demonstrated between these emotional problems and mean labor time, difficulty in labor, and problems in nursing. The pregnant woman's statements about her desire to be pregnant and her maternal feelings were correlated inversely with the degree of gastrointestinal upset during pregnancy.

There is an interesting relationship demonstrated between nausea and psychological variables. A certain amount of morning sickness is correlated with pregnancy, and is expected because of a physical change. However, nausea is also reflective of a woman saying to herself "yes I'm pregnant. See, I'm nauseous." It can express a fulfilling of a cultural expectancy and an inner acknowledgment and acceptance of the pregnancy. Beyond that point, though, when the nausea travels into the later trimester, other factors might be involved. It might be reflective of some kind of psychological conflict, at times interpreted as a wish to "rid" oneself of the child, to "expel it." Grimm & Mann (1962), used the Rorschach and reported that habitual aborters, women who obviously could not "retain" or "hold onto" the fetus, had poorer emotional controls and were more dependent on their mothers than nonhabitual abortors. Davids & Devault (1960) use of selected cards of the Thematic Apperception Test reported an "alienation syndrome," in women with obstetric complications in labor and delivery. He found that egocentricity, pessimism, resentment, and undue hostility was accompanied by considerable withdrawal and pessimism with relationship to the future child. Further research has demonstrated that pregnancy is accompanied by a high degree of manifest anxiety in those women who had abnormal deliveries, prolonged labor time, and abnormal weight gain during the pregnancy. All of these findings and correlations must, of course, be interpreted cautiously with full regard to the possible organic substratum that might exist in these conditions.

A later investigation (Zuckerberg, 1972) explored the relationship between the extreme incidence of certain body symptom complexes during pregnancy and relatively unconscious conflict or acceptance concerning the assumption of the maternal role as well as consciously expressed attitudes toward pregnancy and feminine role function. Specifically, these attitude factors were (1) desire for the pregnancy, (2) attitudes toward labor and delivery, (3) worry with regard to pregnancy and childbirth, (4) marital satisfaction, and (5) dependency in assumption of the sick role. The consistency, or the lack of, between consciously expressed attitudes and unconscious conflict as expressed in structured fantasy was studied in 36 white, native-born, married primigravidas. A clinical analysis of the fantasy responses to a specially devised Pregnancy TAT pointed to the following conflict areas: (1) body image problems; (2) feared loss of dependency associated with the assumption of the maternal role; (3) separation fears associated with delivery; (4) hostility toward the impregnating male and a wish-fear dilemma associated with possible abandonment; (5) concerns about maternal adequacy; (6) role conflict with respect to changes in life-style; and (7) concerns about self-representation.

Body image problems were associated with the acceptance of the physical changes involved in pregnancy, and were accompanied by fears of body damage and vulnerability. That all women are concerned about their body image changes during pregnancy may be mentioned here. The judged evaluation of the PTAT prints indicated that the card depicting the pregnant woman looking at her reflection is by far the most conflicted. This statistic was consistent with Fisher's (1970) research which found that body penetration scores of women during pregnancy increased considerably and that concern about bodily vulnerability is prominent during pregnancy. (This concern decreases after delivery has been successfully completed.) One can tentatively conclude, on the basis of this small sample, that body changes, body awareness, and sexual role attitudes toward the body, i.e., the body as a source of narcissistic pride and injury, is a significant, affective-cognitive core of feminine role conflict. Further, women's feelings, attitudes, and cognitions toward it are markedly conflicted. There also may be a feeling that the body is harboring something that drains the woman, that it is harboring something that is growing without the woman's control or is unknown. All of these states may be accompanied by anxiety and concomitant "warning signals" or may be successfully worked through.

There was feared loss of dependency associated with the assumption of the maternal role. This may involve the fantasized or real loss of supplies from the husband, mother, or father. Transition to motherhood involves becoming an adult, involving, in turn, loss of dependency relationships. One becomes mother, a parent, and accepts, hopefully, in turn, the dependent state of the child. In this process, the woman is hopefully resolving her own dependencies, sometimes through residual identification with the child. There were separation fears associated with delivery. Fears related to being "put out" and the loss of control this entails.

Hostility toward the impregnating male and a wish-fear dilemma was associated with possible abandonment. Many women fear that after giving birth, the husband will desert them. This was a common fear, and most of the time unconscious. When asked "do you worry about him deserting you?" the woman's response would probably be "Oh, no, he'll never do that." But it was an unconscious, repetitive concern as demonstrated in the PTAT stories. One might think, "Well, why do you wish that?" There is conflict about childbearing, and if there is hostility toward the man, perhaps regarding the pregnancy, or his behavior toward the pregnancy, then sometimes a woman might wish unconsciously "I wish he'd go; I wish I could get rid of him." This wish, of course, is accompanied by the fear "If he does, what will I do? I'll be all alone." So it's a wish-fear dilemma relating to the possibility of desertion. Other wish-fear dilemmas may also be expressed but are derived from more deep-seated unconscious material. Also, intrapsychically and developmentally, there is a wish and a fear dilemma having to do with losing one's mother; you want and you fear losing her. On an ego level, you are motivated to accomplish the developmental task of pregnancy and birth, to proceed into adulthood, yet the loss of dependency and the possible abandonment that may come with it is feared. There are dreams about the mother leaving the hospital as the baby comes in; clear dreams about losing the mother and gaining the child as mother; and fear on an oedipal level. If you are successful in having a baby, then there is a fear of abandonment from the mother in the sense of surpassing her. This may be accompanied by guilt and fears of retaliation. The fear of abandonment and the wishes about it run through all levels of development: from oral, having to do with loss of supplies, to anal issues, having to do with control, to the oedipal, which has to do with the loss of the oedipal father and the creation of the father in the husband and the loss of the mother stepping over into the mother's shoes, and the murderous wishes toward the mother that may be involved.

There are general concerns about adequacy as a mother and fantasies about inner emptiness with regard to one's own inner resources and maternal identifications. Ego concerns about adequacy as a mother can be stated as simply "Will I be able to do it?" A lot of working women state "How can I pull this together? Will I be able to organize my time? Who's going to babysit?" These general life concerns, reality factors that are present in the stories may affect the course of pregnancy. Adequacy is also involved in the ability to accept the fetus once it is born as separate from the self. One 60-year-old psychotherapy patient still talks about her children, then over 30-years-old, as babies. This woman, in part, failed to accomplish the task of individuation from her own children. In pregnancy, birth becomes the initial rehearsal for this; the at times experienced "blissful" state of symbiotic oneness with the baby inside must be accepted as lost. There are role conflict issues now with regard to changes in life-style. What does it mean not to work? What do you have to give up? Is it an interruption? What are the real or fantasized losses involved? What are the identity losses? These are issues many women are struggling with today, and talk about initially in counseling sessions. There is, at times, resentment or ambivalence about having to give up one's own autonomy. The conflict may involve loss of independence, leaving behind of gratifying ego supplies, and questions of cultural pressures. Of course, the degree to which all of this is felt depends upon intrapsychic and marital issues.

There is concern about how others, such as peers, family, and members of the older generation view the pregnant woman: "Am I hurting anybody by becoming pregnant?" "Does my husband still think I am desirable?" "What is my mother going to think of me as a mother?" "How do I view myself now?" All of these questions reflect changes in one's self-representation and how one experiences oneself as being viewed by others. The woman who has dependency problems and individuation conflicts will probably be more concerned about what others think. How others view us is a part of our self-esteem and identity. There are those women who care more about what the next person thinks than what they think of themselves. With respect to the above conflicts, it was not the clear absence or presence of the conflicts that discriminated the population, but rather the extent of them and the way in which they were handled. This concerns quality of conflict resolution as well as quantity. In this study, further findings indicated that *when there was a discrepancy between conscious and unconscious attitudes, somatic symptoms occurred with the greatest frequency, and excessive worry was high.* For example, those women who denied conflict through excessively positive attitudes toward pregnancy, and who demonstrated on the PTAT considerable unconscious conflict suffered most from bodily symptoms.

CONCLUSION

To the extent that pregnancy is an experience that expresses a relatively conflict-free, integral life-extension wish and is an affirmation of the marital bond, then the pregnancy experience will probably be benign, integrative, and therapeutic. Women who accomplish this developmental task can come out stronger, more integrated, healthier, and more mature, with or without counseling. It can be, indeed, a reintegrative time for a woman, a time of tremendous gratification, and the problems can be seen as developmental challenges rather than as pathologic. To the extent that pregnancy serves to camouflage a conflict-laden marriage ("We'll keep it together by having a child.") or through denial, maintain a kind of pseudosecurity ("Having a child means we're stable, we're adult."), if it is used to reenact or through acting out, repair unresolved mother-daughter conflicts ("Now she'll respect me."), then the experience, like any other overdetermined life event, will probably be problematic. Undoubtedly, when all goes well, there are multiple positive outcomes. With bearing a child can come a source of self-esteem through generativity, through the assumption of an adult role, and can be accompanied by pride and a feeling of competency. There are examples of positive feelings that women experience and talk about, states of feeling "queenly" after birth, more womanly, and feminine as a mother. It can be a beautiful time. With it comes the opportunity to form a unique mothering identity, an identity separate from one's own mother; with it comes the opportunity for intimacy and sharing within the marital bond. Again, if it goes well, the marriage is better than it ever was. It is richer for there is a sense that the couple has gone through something together and come out of it stronger, perhaps more adult. In this day of merging male-female responsibilities and role identifications (and even the usurping of parental roles by professionals), there are a group of women and men who desire to reinstate a belief system in family and marriage, to guide the future generation with the understandable hope of some kind of personal continuity through children, to reinstate male-female differences, and to affirm the woman's privileged capacity to bear children. This takes hard work and a willingness to forego the novelty, excitement, and change that comes with transitional relationships for the opportunity to maintain a constant continuing relationship that extends into more than the present and helps create a future.

Having a child can indeed be a means of repair of correcting the pain of our own childhood; if we are aware of it, there is untold satisfaction that comes from *not* repeating what is so very often repeated in the tragicomic human condition. Through our children we can hope to instill, within limits, what we found missing in our own upbringing.

Any conflict or ambivalence that is felt during pregnancy is more often than not met with intense feelings of shame and guilt, and sometimes if the guilt is severe enough, an inner feeling of malevolence, for if the woman has any attachment at all to implicit societal expectations and ideals, she will expect of herself to be welcoming her future child. Not only will the conflict be experienced between herself and the pregnancy condition, but between herself and birth and delivery; between herself and the future child, who may become the target of countless projections and distortions; between herself and her husband; between herself and the marital bond; between herself and her nuclear family. Of course, like any life event that involves change and growth, it is going to be imbedded in some measure of ambivalence. There is always a loss of autonomy and increase in the symbiotic pull, which depending upon the mother, may feel comfortable or not in the beginning relationship to the infant. There is always some financial strain, and, in the first year, especially, there is always for the mother decreased ties to the outer world. But, no matter how ambivalent, or even at times deeply resentful toward her child, there is always some part of her that wants to meet this new human being as accepted in health.

There appears to be some existential core problems involving transition from self to other, the beginning and extension of a future through a child as an extension of oneself, from self-time to child-time. There may be an experiencing of time slowing down, of time being shaped by the steady monitoring of a child's growth. There may be a feeling of aloneness and loneliness, because, after all, the ultimate responsibility does lie with the mother, or, at least, it is felt that way.

Klein et al. (1950) found a high incidence of irrational anxieties during pregnancy. Concern about death of self was frequently expressed despite the fact that maternal and fetal death rate in pregnancy and delivery is practically negligible. Besides the possibility of underlying rage that might be directed against the self or child, and manifest in this fear, there may be also a possible concern about self survival in a more basic sense, i.e., a concern about one's own inner resources, supplies, and separateness. And this might be quite usual in the conflicts that occur during the time of pregnancy.

A woman's attitudes and feelings toward pregnancy are complex. If a "bad" pregnancy can be predicted on the basis of a psychological check-up with attention to warning signals, then psychological guidance and support can possibly be given. Such an intervention would not only help in the lessening of somatic problems but may actually decrease the incidence of abnormal births, spontaneous abortions, and postpartum depressions. More importantly, a positively experienced, supported pregnancy might help to encourage a relatively successful early mother–child interaction.

The option for a woman in conflict over her pregnancy is

now either to carry to term or to seek an abortion. Perhaps with some psychological understanding, the complexities of acceptance or rejection of the child can be explored and the choices increased for the woman bearing a child. It is obvious to the author that the psychological repercussions of intentional abortion are not well understood and that such a method of dealing with this problem is frequently far from being therapeutic for the woman involved, or, in fact, the correct decision.

The major risks of pregnancy today are no longer medical, but psychological. The essential ingredients of sexual identity are being questioned and reevaluated. In times of transitional crisis, there can be a reawakening to some of these issues and a sensitizing to the psychological joys and issues involved in making this transition from self to other.

Suggested Plan of Intervention

This notion can be implemented into a plan of focused intervention with prevention of pathologic maternal-child conflicts as the aim. The following model is in progress:[2]

1. A medical-psychological team approach may be implemented during early pregnancy with follow-up throughout the first year postpartum. The psychologist would act with the obstetrician as an ongoing psychological consultant. The woman is encouraged to talk to the psychologist in the beginning of her pregnancy and this would be considered routine, a "psychological check-up," not reserved for serious problems alone, but as a standard and expected part of the total medical and psychological care.

[2]The PSYCHOLOGICAL CONSULTATION SERVICE FOR PARENTS AND PERSPECTIVE PARENTS, founded by Joan Offerman–Zuckerberg, has been established with this model in mind.

2. The psychologist would assess at this point the degree of severity of conflicts and, where indicated, would be available to follow a short-term psychotherapeutic approach with the woman.
3. In the third trimester, all women would be encouraged to speak to the psychologist concerning their expectations, fears, hopes, and concerns regarding pregnancy.
4. In the hospital, the psychologist would be available to the mother for counseling. The immediate postpartum period is an especially excellent time for therapeutic intervention.
5. During the first year of early mothering, the psychologist would be available for questions and would remain sensitive to and helpful about the developmental changes that occur in the mother during this transitional time.
6. During the entire course of pregnancy and early maternal care, if the husband could and would want to respond to these services and participate in them, he would be urged and encouraged, and it would be considered fundamentally important to the effectiveness of the total program.

It is the author's contention that this program could be considered an effective tool in the prevention of human psychopathology. The stubborn obstacles would be in the area of encouraging active questioning in the couple, sensitivity on the part of the medical team, and a willingness on the part of both parent and professional to share information and control. This program requires interdisciplinary effort and a flexible attitude to professional boundaries.

Review of Physical Warning Signals

1. Habitual abortion.
2. Hypertension, which would be of particular impor-

tance psychologically, if there was no history for this prior to pregnancy.

3. Undue nausea—a complete absence of nausea may indicate denial of the pregnancy. Nausea extending through the 3rd or 4th month may indicate psychic ambivalence. Some nausea may indicate cultural and individual acceptance and recognition.

4. Inappropriate weight gain—an unusual reliance on food consumption during this time may indicate inner feelings of depletion, emptiness, conflict, and emotional hunger.

5. Unusual and vague aches, cramps, and pains in the genital area. Pains in this area, as it is the site of sexual intercourse, may be "body language" statements regarding conflicts concerning pregnancy and childbearing, in general.

6. Blushing, flushing, and fainting. This conversion may involve shame regarding pregnancy as a sexual act and denial through fainting.

7. Breathing difficulties. The conversion might be feelings of constriction and suffocation regarding loss of autonomy.

8. Gastrointestinal complaints. The conversion might be "I can't stomach this" or "this tastes bad." These are conflicts regarding incorporation.

9. Circulation problems and general aches and pains may have numerous interpretations, including dependency wishes for attention. "Look how I'm suffering" or a general translation of the feeling "Look how painful this is."

All of these somatic signs lend themselves to multiple interpretations, and to multiple forms of conversion language. The signals mentioned are merely examples of how the language can work and exist along a continuum from normal intensity to distressful.

Review of Psychological Warning Signals

Psychological warning signals are harder to interpret because they are experienced usually in a less focused way, without physical site. As mentioned, all women experience all of these feelings. The degree, duration, and extent of the attending anxiety are what differentiates common signs of developmental stress from what might be a "problem." Examples are:

1. Excessive worries and/or fears regarding damage to self during pregnancy, to future child, to the marriage, and to parents. This might be accompanied by feelings that others might hurt you or are critical of you.
2. Unusual fantasies or thoughts experienced as "out of control" regarding possibly loss of control in pregnancy and childbirth or abandonment from husband and mother.
3. Acute and prolonged separation anxiety manifest in prolonged depression, periods of agitation and depression, chronic marital fighting with a focus on jealousy and abandonment fears, guilt toward one's mother and rekindled ambivalence, regressive "girl-like" behavior, whining, an upsurge of dependent feelings.
4. Loss of emotional responsiveness, feelings of "not feeling," of "being out of it," of "not being myself," of feeling "like I'm watching everyone."
5. Unusual mood swings without source, from extreme lability to periods of withdrawal and hostile silences, angry outbursts without explanation and then, without memory.
6. Resistance to nestbuilding: no effort to select a name, to prepare a room, to order and clean the house, to work on solidifying the marital bond.

Again, all of these emotional warning signals can be expressed in many different forms and are basically individual in expression and nature. It is hoped that when attention is turned to these warning signals, through a psychological check-up, we can then more effectively initiate a program in the primary prevention of family pathology and facilitate more generally, a healthy transition into parenthood.

REFERENCES

Davids, A., & Devault, S. Use of the TAT and human figure drawings in research on personality, pregnancy and perception. *Journal of Projective Techniques,* 1960, *24,* 362–365.

Fischer, S. *Body experiences in fantasy and behavior.* New York: Appelton, 1970.

Grimm, E. R. Psychological and social factors in pregnancy, delivery and outcome, in S. A. Richardson & A. Guttmacher (eds), *Childbearing: its social and psychological aspects.* Baltimore: Williams & Wilkins, 1967.

Grimm, E. R., & Mann, E. C. Psychological investigation of habitual abortions. *Psychosomatic Medicine,* 1962, *14,* 369–378.

Heinstein, M. Expressed attitudes and feelings of pregnant women. *Merrill-Palmer Quarterly,* 1967, *13,* 217–236.

Klein, H. R., Potter, J. W., & Dyk, B. *Anxiety in pregnancy and childbirth.* New York: Paul P. Halber, 1950.

Knobel, M. Psicoteropia preventiva en el embarazo. Presentado of VII Congreso Internacional de Psicoterapia, Wiesbaden, Argosto 25, 1967.

Loftus, T. A. Behavioral and psychoanalytic aspects of anovulatory and amenorrhea. *Journal of Fertility and Sterility,* 1962, *13,* 1.

Tanzer, D. W. Psychology of pregnancy and childbirth. Unpublished doctoral dissertation, 1967.

Wittkower, L. A global survey of psychosomatic medicine. *Psychosomatic Medicine,* 1969, *3,* 722–737.

Zuckerberg, J. An exploration into feminine role conflict and body symptomatology in pregnancy. Unpublished doctoral dissertation, 1972.

BIBLIOGRAPHY

Alexander, F. *Psychosomatic Medicine.* New York: Norton, 1950.

Ballou, J. W. *The psychology of pregnancy.* Lexington, Ma.: D.C. Heath, 1978.

Benedek, T. The psychosomatic implications of the primary unit: mother-child. *American Journal of Orthopsychiatry,* 1949, *19,* 642.

Benedek, T. *Psychosexual tendencies in women.* New York: Ronald Press, 1952.

Benedek, T. The psychoobiology of pregnancy, in Anthony, E. J. & Benedek, T. (eds). *Parenthood: its psychology and psychopathology.* Boston: Little Brown, 1970.

Bibring, G. Some considerations of the psychological processes in pregnancy. *The Psychoanalytic Study of the Child,* 1959, *14,* 113–121.

Bibring, G. A study of the psychological processes in pregnancy and of the earliest mother-child relationship. *The Psychoanalytic Study of the Child,* 1961, *16,* 9–72.

Colman, A. *First baby group. An investigation into the psychology of pregnancy and mothering.* Unpublished, 1966.

Davids, A., Holden, R., & Gray, G. Maternal anxiety during pregnancy and adequacy of mother and child adjustment eight months following birth. *Child Development,* 1963, *34,* 993–1002.

Deutsch, H. *Psychology of Women* (Vols. 1 & 2). New York: Grune & Stratton, 1944, 1945.

Dunbar, F. Emotional factors in spontaneous abortion. In *Psychosomatic obstetrics, gynecology and endocrinology.* Chas. C. Thomas, Springfield, Ill. 1963.

Frankle, A. H. Psychometric investigation of the relationship between emotional repression and the occurrence of psychosomatic symptoms, *Psychosomatic Medicine,* 1952, *15,* 253–255.

Grinkler, R. R. *Psychosomatic research.* New York: Norton, 1953.

Grimm, E. R., & Venet, R. The role of emotional adjustment and attitudes in pregnant women. *Psychosomatic Medicine,* 1966, *28* (1), 34–49.

Knobel, M., & Vigneau, M. Technica Projectiva para el estudio de la person-alidad de la mayer embrarazada. *Archivos de Criminologia Nuevo Psy-chiatria - Diciplenas Conexas,* 1967, *15,* 43–65.

McDonald, R. L. Fantasy and the outcome of pregnancy. *Archives of General Psychiatrics,* 1965, *12,* 602.

McDonald, R. L., & Christakos, A. C. Relationship of emotional adjustment during pregnancy and obstretical complications. *American Journal of Obstetrics and Gynecology,* 1962, *64,* 341.

Menninger, C. The emotional factors in pregnancy. *Bulletin of the Menninger Clinic,* 1943, *7,* 15–24.

Robertson, G. G. Nausea and vomiting of pregnancy. *Lancet,* 1946, *2,* 336.

Rosen, S. Emotional factors in nausea and vomiting of pregnancy. *Psychiatry Quarterly,* 1955, *29,* 621.

chapter 10

PSYCHOTHERAPY WITH PREGNANT WOMEN

Joan Raphael-Leff

At the core of woman lies a secret inner chamber that is the center of life. It lies dormant, fallow, and unknowable during all the years of her childhood until, in adolescence, it awakens sending monthly reminders of its existence, waiting empty and unfulfilled. Then the void is filled and closes around a fertilized seed of future life. Whatever its fate, the process is irreversible. The mystery begins to unfold and the woman is in touch with the primordial forces of pregnancy existing since time immemorial.

A number of authorities have recognized pregnancy as a *normal transitional crisis* (Benedek, 1970; Bibring et al; 1959, 1961; Caplan, 1959; Deutsch, 1947; Hanford, 1968; Rapoport, 1963) and have stressed the profound emotional disequilibrium of the pregnant woman and her vulnerability to psychological disturbances. The following have been found to be widespread in normal antenatal clinic populations: anxiety (Jarrahi-Zadeh

The women quoted were in individual or group psychotherapy with the author. Names were changed to ensure confidentiality.

et al; 1964; Klein et al., 1950); depression (Jarrahi-Zadeh et al., 1964; Kumar & Robson, 1978); worry, mood lability, insomnia, and impaired cognitive functioning (Jarrahi-Zadeh et al., 1964); stress and emotional conflicts (Hanford, 1968); severe disturbances of thought and behavior, premonitions, magical thinking, paranoid and depressive reactions (Bibring, 1959); regressive shifts and emergence of earlier behavior patterns, attitudes, conflicts, and increased dependency needs (Bibring et al., 1961; Pines 1972; Rapoport 1963; Wenner et al., 1964).

Because the transitional crisis of pregnancy and childbirth involves widespread psychological changes and emotional upheavals, a reappraisal and redefinition of identity is necessitated, particularly in the first pregnancy. Although western woman is as deeply affected by this crisis as are many of her counterparts in traditional societies, she finds herself having to face this uncharted critical phase as an individual, without any of the traditional rituals which serve as an outlet for anxiety and a framework for resolving conflicts and complex feelings.

In traditional societies, the pregnant woman is protected by the initiated, encircled throughout her inner journey into the vortex of myths, magic, and metaphors. Society at large recognizes the significance of the critical phase she has entered and provides her with a framework of rituals, ceremonies, and concepts which enable her to express, channel, and master the complex emotional experiences of this transitional period.

The great anthropologist Malinowski (1955) states that in most cultures

> "the physiological phases of human life, and above all, its crises, such as conception, pregnancy, birth, puberty, marriage and death form the nuclei of numerous rites and beliefs. Thus beliefs about conception, such as that in reincarnation, spirit-entry, magical impregnation, exist in one form or another in almost every tribe, and they are often associated with rites and observances. During pregnancy the expectant mother has to keep certain taboos and undergo ceremonies, and her husband shares at times in both. At birth, before and after, there are various

magical rites to prevent dangers and undo sorcery, ceremonies
of purification, communal rejoicings and acts of presentation of
the newborn to higher powers or to the community (p. 37).

In the western world, with the development of urban technological societies, traditional rituals have tended to fade away
although some still persist in religious communities.* However,
there is a "widespread explicit rejection of rituals as such"
(Douglas, 1973, p. 19) despite the relatively unchanged nature
of these critical events.

Modern medical science has inaugurated an age of increased physical safety for the pregnant woman and her baby.
However the caring professions have sorely neglected her emotional and psychological needs at this time. In view of the
limited therapeutic resources available, and the ubiquitous nature of pregnancy, it is worth considering alternative forms of
care which represent an efficient use of resources. These may
include psychotherapeutic groups, self-help discussion groups,
groups exploring the emotions of pregnancy attached to childbirth education classes, continuous ante- and postnatal support
groups run by health care professionals in clinics, and the enlistment of community support: surrogate grandmothers, a befriending network of pregnant women, or mothers of young
babies, etc. The only prerequisite for group leaders (other than
general mental health) is that they should have experienced a
full-term pregnancy.

Although most women eventually achieve the "maturational integration" (Bibring, 1959) that their new identity necessitates, there are some women who are particularly liable to
succumb to the disturbances of this period. A woman at risk
requires *individualized attention* "as she might need a blood

---

*Within the Jewish faith, for example, a network of beliefs and customs
are available to mark these *rites de passage*. These are guidelines relating to
sex and conception, prayers following childbirth, rituals of circumcision, and
even the still practiced ancient rite of the "Redemption of the Firstborn."

transfusion or some other emergency measure to carry her through the crisis of pregnancy and delivery" (Wenner et al., 1964, p. 409). Clearly, ill adjustment to pregnancy does not merely affect the pregnant woman's psychic health but is likely to affect the physical welfare of the fetus (James, 1969), the course of the pregnancy and labor (Breen 1975; Davids et al., 1961; Hanford 1968; Klein et al., 1950), and of course, the future stability of the mother and emotional development of the infant.

WOMEN AT RISK

Double Crisis

These are the women who, in addition to the major demands of pregnancy, are having to contend with other, at times, conflicting transitional crises. Thus, the adolescent primigrava has a great deal of upheaval. Similarly, widowhood coinciding with pregnancy involves a double crisis adjustment, as do elderly primagrava (35 plus with the menopause in sight), diabetic or chronically physically ill women, and women with preexisting psychiatric illness.

Life events Occurring During Pregnancy

Sudden, usually unforseen and/or untimely happenings which necessitate an alteration in psychosocial adjustment are called *life events*. These, like the crises above, interrupt the natural emotional process of pregnancy. Additional upheavals and intrusive external stimuli are imposed. However, whereas the crises above were "chronic" and "ongoing," life events may be short-lived and affect the pregnant woman at a tangent, or with less immediacy than the former. Thus, they may include bereavement, loss of job, moving, etc.

The Unsupported Woman

Wenner et al. (1964), Pines (1972), and others have stressed the need of the pregnant woman for a supportive and dependable environment. The absence of a stable sexual partner, marital conflicts, geographical or emotional unavailability of her mother or close friends augur badly during this time of increased dependency and need for reassurance. Marital problems during pregnancy are commonly exacerbated by emotional changes in the wife, mood swings, introversion, irritability, extreme sensitivity or tiredness, and changes in her sexual patterns (Caplan, 1959). In addition to these sudden inexplicable changes, it is very likely that the husband feels left out of the exciting process of creativity, set aside like a drone in the beehive whereas the wife and baby are now the focus of attention. Many of these complaints can be anticipated and explained as temporary and necessary adjustments of the woman to her "crisis," but ongoing support still may be indicated.

The unsupported single pregnant woman is likely to have conceived "as part of a process seeking to resolve or diminish a state of anxiety stemming from some neurosis or source of conflict" (Greenberg et al., 1959, p. 296). One such possibility are women, particularly sensitive to separations, who become pregnant following a loss, and use the pregnancy to reenact the separation by placing their infants for adoption. These, and other women who intend having their babies adopted, are in need of special attention due to their double tasks of sustaining life and mourning the loss of the baby. The unsupported single mother is particularly at risk after the birth of the baby when all the functions of mothering and fathering fall upon her, without the care of a mothering figure for herself. Good mothering appears to necessitate a hierarchy of caring or "three generational parenting" (Pines, 1978a) and when absent in the natural environment should be supplemented by health care workers.

Previous Abortion, Stillbirth, or Infant with Congenital Abnormalities

A history of pregnancies that did not bear the fruit of a live, healthy child raises the possibility of unresolved mourning. Emotional links with previous pregnancies are revived during each subsequent one and old conflicts may fester in the context of the new. Thus, Kumar and Robson (1978) found a link in primiparas between previous abortion and current depression during pregnancy, and intensification of anxieties about fetal abnormalities in these women, suggesting fear of punishment and retribution. These were not found in expectant mothers who had had miscarriages. Women who are ambivalent about their pregnancies and actually consider abortion are more likely to be depressed during the first trimester and in the first few months after the baby is born. (Kumar & Robson, personal communication). Similarly, feelings of shame, guilt, horror, and grief surrounding an earlier stillbirth may be revived during pregnancy, coupled with fears and conflictual feelings about the survival of the present fetus. (Lewis, 1976) In addition to therapeutic intervention during subsequent pregnancies, there is clearly a need to provide special psychological care for women undergoing termination. Needless to say, women who have given birth to a child with congenital abnormalities need help during subsequent pregnancies.

Anorexia Nervosa and Compulsive Eating Patterns

Women with a past history of anorexia or with current patterns of compulsive eating have problems regarding their body image, the representation of boundaries between their internal and external worlds, and fantasies about the content or emptiness within. These are exacerbated during pregnancy, as are conflicts regarding femininity and adulthood often symbolized by earlier abnormal cessation of menstruation, disguised breast development within body fat, and so on. In addition to therapeutic intervention during and possibly after pregnancy, these women require special consultations with and sensitive surveillance by a nutritionist or dietitian to ensure a rational intake of the necessary nutrients. Obviously, *pseudocyesis* (false pregnancy) must be treated very seriously upon discovery and individual psychotherapy offered without delay.

Women in a "Feminine Revolt"

This refers to women who cannot easily accept their identity as feminine. It is possible to distinguish two groups among these women. First are those who are involved in a revolt against their own mothers, and particularly against the image of the *powerful mother* of infancy and early childhood. This "need to detach oneself from the primal omnipotent mother by denying her faculties, her (reproductive) organs and her specifically feminine features and by investing in the father, seems to be a need which both sexes share" during their childhood (Chassguet-Smirgel, 1976, p. 284). Some girls, however, take this wish to break away to great extremes (possibly due to blaming her lack of penis onto her "castrating" mother) (Lampl de Groot, 1933) projecting all the mother's power onto the father, his penis, male activities, and masculine identity thereby denuding the mother of anything valuable to offer her, and herself of her own feminine identity. If she becomes pregnant, such a woman has no benevolent maternal image to call upon, few positive feminine resources within her own self-representation, and, at times, an active abhorrence of her own position as fertile, pregnant, and femininely creative. Clearly, she would also have severe doubts about her own capacity to become a good mother and fear retaliation for usurping her originally powerful mother.

Second, the other group consists of women who have not achieved separation from a possibly overinvolved and/or needy mother, seen as a victim of male tyranization or neglect. This type of woman tends to dissipate her energies in hating men and her father in particular, blaming him for "castrating" her mother and herself, while identifying femininity with the bro-kendown, passive, and *powerless mother.* During pregnancy, she is filled with hatred for her sexual partner and his represen-tation within her womb, and has grave doubts about her ability to cope as a future mother, especially to a male child. A varia-tion on this pattern is discussed by Balint (1972). These are the women who maintain their original active loving relationship with their early mothers who were invariably depressed or withdrawn. Although forming relationships with men in later life and enjoying their own feminine bodies, they remain in-wardly preoccupied with women and the need to "satisfy" them, and maintain their own femininity at the price of catering to other women's needs in an effort to ward off their envy. All of these women are particularly vulnerable during pregnancy and are liable, if untreated, to have a *puerperal breakdown* after the birth, related to problems of masculine identification or feminine identity (Hayman, 1962; Lomas, 1960)

Pregnancy Following "Functional Sterility"

Difficulties in conceiving due to psychogenic factors are not necessarily fully resolved when pregnancy occurs. The deep-seated anxieties about the dangers inherent in fertility, procreation, and motherhood may cause great distortions in the woman's relationship to her fetus, and later to her baby.

MATURATIONAL STAGES OF PREGNANCY AND CONCOMITANT THERAPEUTIC TASKS

Pregnancy may be subdivided into three basic stages: *The first stage,* lasting from awareness of conception until the first felt movements of the fetus, necessitates adjustment to a dra-matic change in *self-image.* Whatever the outcome, the alteration is irreversible, a point of no return (Caplan, 1959; Erikson, 1964; Pines, 1972) implying "the end of the woman as an independent single unit and the beginning of an unalterable and irrevocable mother-child relationship" (Pines, 1972, p. 333).

However wanted the pregnancy, this stage will involve coming to terms with the inevitable negative and conflictual feelings towards the baby (Hanford, 1968) and will necessitate an increased emotional investment in the "foreign body" making it into an *integral part* of her own being (Bibring et al., 1961; Chertok, 1966; Benedek, 1970; Deutsch, 1947; Pines, 1972).

The discovery of pregnancy also involves an adjustment to a new and rapidly changing *body image*. The primagravida must expand her physical consciousness to include the hitherto dormant and unexplored interior of her womb, as upon losing her virginity she had to encompass her semi mysterious vagina. (see Chassguet-Smirgel, 1976; Deutsch, 1925; Fast, 1978; Freud, 1925; Gillespie, 1975; Horney, 1926; Jaffe, 1968; Jacobson, 1968; Kestenberg, 1968; Klein, 1932; Moore, 1968, 1976; on the controversy of relative ignorance versus innate knowledge of the vagina). Unfortunately, in addition to her inner space being taken over and defined by an "interloper," the newly pregnant woman, often finds it externally invaded by detached probing fingers; unprefaced introduction of cold, duck-billed instruments; and sudden bright lights shone up her dark vagina during internal medical examinations. The adjustment to a new body image, also include tender and enlarging breasts, and rapid expansion of body boundaries, reviving adolescent conflicts and stresses. But most of all, the expectant mother must come to terms with the strange *"two-in-one"* phenomena, the weird experience of two people in one body. As one patient stated: "Haven't got your body for your sole occupation any more—got somebody else down there—bloody cheek! . . . it would be so nice to have my body back under my control, could drink, smoke wear nice clothes" . . . (Janet).

Pregnancy forms a "visible manifestation to the outside world" of having had a sexual relationship (Pines, 1972, p. 334) as well as carrying in the womb a tangible physical and psychic representation of her sexual partner (Deutsch, 1947). This necessitates further expansion and intergration of her feminine identity and reassessment of her relationship with her man (shift from two-fold "dyadic" relationship to "triadic" unit to include the baby [Breen, 1975]). In addition, she undergoes a reactivation of her archaic relationship to her own mother, often accompanied by revival of childhood envies and jealousies, shame and guilt, as well as fears of punishment for "usurping" or surpassing her mother. These feelings sometimes lead to an inability to tell her parents that she is pregnant. "I'm afraid to tell them—they'll want to take it away" (Carol); "destroy it by remote control" (Lucy); "steal it back" (Mary). In order to become a well-adjusted mother herself, she must also engage in adaptive modifications to her concept of "motherliness" based on often idealized or denigrated identifications with her early mother (Breen, 1975) and come to terms with her real mother, thus enabling herself to become a "good enough" mother (Winnicott, 1958).

This first stage involves a marked regression to *oral preoccupations* and early magical ideas about conception being due to eating or swallowing something (Freud, 1908). During this period, physical symptoms that occur may take on symbolic meanings. For example, nausea and vomiting may express a protest against the intruder or unconscious rejection of the feminine role (Menninger, 1943). Food cravings also often are symbolic, for example women desire grains and seeds, womb-shaped pears, spices, and cucumbers signifying "reincorporation" and "affirmation of fecundation" (Deutsch, 1950). Also common are fantasies of being "sucked dry" or "sapped" by the fetus: "I feel I've been taken over by a being from outer space —a Martian or something who is using my body—feeding off it and leaving me exhausted . . . I've always had perfect teeth, but now my dentist tells me I need 4 fillings!" (Rachel)

The second stage of pregnancy is heralded by the quickening which emphasizes both the separate nature of the fetus and the uncontrollable, inexorable process of development which the pregnant woman can scarcely influence, but has to actively tolerate: "This is beyond my control. I've never had to face such a prolonged period of uncertainty before" (Rachel). Indeed, there is perhaps no other human endeavor in which one individual invests her resources so generously, so totally emotionally and bodily, with so long-term a commitment and so very little knowledge of the successful outcome and final "product"! (This explains why any "message from the interior" such as a blood test results or information from an ultrasound scan become so highly valued).

During this stage, "the psychic hygiene of pregnancy must aim at making the child more and more of an object (i.e. whole person) so that delivery does not have the effect of a painful separation from a part of the ego, and a distinctive psychic loss" (Deutsch, 1947, p. 135). I have found that expectant mothers initiate verbal communication with the fetus during this stage, and increase the nonverbal contact by singing to the fetus, stroking, patting, cradling, smacking(!) it. These are undoubtedly indications of the process of becoming "familiar" with the fetus, filling the uncertainty with a face, gender, fantasy personality, and, often, features and a name, somewhat like the development of an "imaginary friend" in childhood. The process of giving the baby a reality, however, brings home the inevitability of the separation which must come about with birth accompanied by mixed feelings of wanting to "meet" yet retain the inner friend: "She was a fantastic companion. I was always talking to her, messing about as if she was outside, but when she was being born, I got so angry with her and started shouting: 'get back! Please go back inside!' " (This is Valerie talking about a previous pregnancy.) Simultaneously, there is a reemergence of old feelings related to the toilet-training era, anxieties about bodily control, retention, or expulsion of feces. At times the fetus is likened to a stool, based on early magical equations of "breast-womb-intestine-feces-baby" (Jacobson, 1936) or "motion-gift-penis-child" (Abraham, 1920; Freud, 1917). Also evident, are residues of primitive notions of bisexuality (i.e., both sexes have penis and can give birth, (Freud, 1908; Fast, 1978). To some women, the fetus may begin to represent an internal penis, compensating her for her original pain upon her discovery of sexual differences (Chasseguet-Smirgel, 1976). The sperm that has been retained and "grows" in the womb, moving of its own accord, gives some women a fantasy of having gained masculine powers. These mothers-to-be may see their fetus as male and attribute heroic and messianic capacities to their unborn child. A resolution of these fantasies before the birth is vital to a realistic mother–child relationship after the birth.

Oral fantasies remain active during this stage, likening the fetus to "a great big ravenous mouth eating up" the mother's insides (Ruth); or "greedily sucking milk" from the "internal breasts" (Mary); and there is a magical preoccupation with nutrition: "feeding the baby wholesome foods to pacify its anger" (Helen); "drinking loads of milk so as not to run dry"; (Mary); eating or avoiding certain foods which have symbolic connotations: "strawberries might produce naevi" (Pines, 1972, p. 336); "eating dates will bring a boy" (Jewish-Moroccan belief); "eating sharp foods strengthens the fetus" (Polish superstition).

A preoccupation common to all women during the second stage of pregnancy is whether or not the baby will be normal. Often, women are convinced that they will have a miscarriage or that the baby will be deformed or be stillborn due to a primitive belief in Fate that will finally punish them for old sins and present good fortune, and above all retribution for the guilty crime of wanting to take mother's place. Constant active vigilance over the fetus and superstitious precautions are taken to avoid fate. It is at this time that "the 'secret society of women' with its rituals and old wives' tales can be observed and where men are sometimes regarded as intruders capable of harming the child" (Pines, 1972, p. 336). Often accompanied by avoidance of sexual intercourse, a typical fantasy at this time is that of the *immaculate conception*. Betty, an unmarried filmscript writer, 16 weeks pregnant, described her decision to conceive:

> "I was in the desert—all around was natural progress surrounded by people having children naturally without the conflicts and doubts that are our currency. Suddenly, on my 31st birthday, I felt so tired of other people's productions—of hoping each film would be important and different; tired of money squabbles, tired of other people sharing or dictating, and above all, tired of discovering on delivery day that it wasn't worth it all. I wanted to do something by myself, alone."

Her feelings about the birth were consistent with this almost immaculate conception, and her desire for this "delivery day" to be her own "special production." Much to the consternation of the hospital staff, she invited six friends from all over the world to come and be present at the birth.

Another reason for refraining from sex at this stage is a fear of harming the baby (related to the notion that sexual activities are dangerous or dirty) or a fantasy that the now "live" (i.e., moving) baby can witness the parental intercourse from within (Abraham, 1923).

Many women relive their own mother's pregnancies at this time, either their own conception and birth, or that of the sibling equivalent to their own current parity. I have called this the *Quaker-Oats phenomena* (Quaker Oats box with a picture of a Quaker holding a Quaker-Oats box with a picture of a Quaker . . .) as it is potentially an eternal reenactment, and frequently referred to as an "infinite regression." It is particularly pertinent in the case of women whose mothers had unusual or morbid experiences during pregnancy and/or childbirth, or gave vivid, lurid, or mystifying accounts of these events, or women whose early identification with their mothers had not been modified while pregnant.

> Lilly was adopted at 3 weeks with no knowledge of her origins. As a child she was haunted by the fear of being infertile because she was adopted. Following her adoptive mother's death of

stomach cancer, Lilly conceived and had two children. Her third pregnancy was unwanted but she did not have an abortion since she felt she owed her life to the fact that her natural mother had not had one. Of this pregnancy she says: "I feel the baby moving in somebody else's womb . . ." "It's as if I'm watching this baby grow in a bottle . . . somebody else is pregnant with this baby. The baby is like a cancerous growth invading my body—going its course, out of my control, without my consent. A baby is like putting a parcel in the post with no address, to see if it will arrive at the correct destination . . ." Thus, she reenacts her biological mother's rejecting pregnancy with herself, as well as her adoptive mother's detached waiting for the baby that will be "delivered," as well as the link with her illness.

The third and final stage of pregnancy is marked by an increased concern about labor, fears of damage, exposure, and separation. Despite fatigue and physical discomfort, "nesting behavior" develops that leads to wallpapering, oven cleaning, floor scrubbing, and polishing. I am again impelled to quote Deutsch's (1947) masterly description of this stage:

> With the increase of bodily discomfort, the ego of a psychically healthy woman becomes gradually weary of the shrinking of her life contents produced by pregnancy and of her exceptional physical and psychic situations. Apparently the merger of extremes —ego and species—cannot be tolerated for a very long time. The relationship with the child is split: the being in the uterus already has his double, who is the subject of all expectations and fantasied wish fulfilments and whose real existence as a distinct person is gradually approaching. With the end of the pregnancy the I-you polarity is simultaneously strengthened, and the psychic management of loving and hostile impulses uses this duality: the enemy must get out in order to reappear as a precious friend in the outside world" (p. 186).

Most writers date this stage rather vaguely towards the end of pregnancy. I have found that the beginning of the third stage can be pinpointed in time. It coincides with the pregnant woman's belief in the viability of the real baby outside her body. Some women place it at 28 weeks, the earliest date of known viability; others at 32 or 36 weeks, when the baby could survive without an incubator. The important factor is that the baby could now do without its "hothouse" mother, and she begins to envisage doing without her seedling. Whereas previously the EDD (expected delivery date) was anticipated with concern about "what if the baby is early?" she now says: "What if it is late." This watershed brings with it a renewed wave of complaints about the physical discomforts of pregnancy (largely absent during the second stage) and many fantasies of regaining ownership of her own body: sleeping on her stomach once more, taking an aspirin, or seeing her toes.

One of the primitive concepts reawakened during pregnancy is that of a *single internal cavity* within the body. Naturally, this involves a confusion between the various elements contained within the stomach, namely, food, fetus, feces, internal organs, urine, amniotic fluid, and milk. One of the secret anxieties of many women is that during childbirth "the baby will pull everything out after it—everything inside will just come spilling out, lungs, liver, even the brains" (Rachel). Later, there might be difficulties in suckling while menstruating or passing the postpartum discharge for fear of "the milk being poisonous" (Rachel). (This must be considered as a possible reason for failure in breastfeeding, and the common coincidence of weaning when periods return).

Another common anxiety relating to childbirth is a fear of the *episiotomy* (a surgical cut in the perineum, often made routinely in hospital to facilitate delivery). This anxiety has the obvious connotations that most minor operations arouse, but at a deeper level fears regarding femininity ("How does one ever make love again without fear of the scar opening?" and the revival of old "castration" anxieties ("It will damage me—like reopening an old wound"). Sometimes there are fantasies of alternative birth channels, for example, a slit in the stomach like the wolf in Red Riding-Hood (Freud, 1908, p. 219). "Birth is so unnatural! That modern medicine should still assume that babies be born rather than removed when ready! The only reason I don't want a cesarean is because I don't want a scar on my stomach" (Helen). Another example is birth "via the navel which comes open" (Freud, 1908). "Sometimes it seems to me that the baby's belly-button is attached to mine inside with the cord so if they (midwives) pulled it the baby would pop out" (Mary) (see also Rosner, 1978). In this stage too, the Quaker Oats syndrome may be seen, specific fears about labor based on accounts of their own or sibling's births. Occasionally, if not worked through during pregnancy, these or reactions against them may actually be reenacted on the delivery table.

The powerful fear of loss of consciousness and its attendant fears of death are common to most women approaching labor. *Fear of death* during or following delivery is very common among contemporary women despite the advances of medicine, the infrequency of complications, and the very active intellectual and physical preparation of many women for the birth itself. This too, is a fear few "enlightened" pregnant women can disclose. Nevertheless, it is persistent despite their dismissing it as ridiculous. Indeed, it is partly due to birth being associated with the primitive elements of blood and pain linked with morbid states. In addition, birth has often been regarded as a magical event, during which the parturient possesses powers that are dangerous to the uninitiated (Benedek 1977). Many pregnant women fear that during labor they will cry out, curse, weep, or scream; that they will lose control and spill out the content of their bodies and minds, reveal their innards and hitherto hidden parts of themselves, deliver dark secrets and be separated from their core. Birth is the prototype of all separations and this, naturally, is a key fear in birth: the mother losing her companion of 9 months and very aware that the child is losing her and the total security of the womb. Some stress that the woman's own birth trauma is mastered "in the actively repeated act of parturition, for to the unconscious carrying and being carried, giving birth and being born, are as identical as giving suck and sucking" (Deutsch, 1925, p. 171).

Another typical anxiety of the pregnant woman is that of

giving birth in the presence of *strangers*. It is curious, how readily we accept that this most intimate of happenings with its accompanying intense emotions should take place in public under the glare of a spotlight. The common experience is that the parturient is merely a laboring vehicle. Far from being recognized as the natural conclusion to a natural process and the final accomplishment following months of anticipation and preparation, few women can even be "brave" enough to take up the gravity-assisted position of squatting, for fear they will disconnect the intravenous drip, disrupt the proceedings or anger the deliverers.

"I really didn't want any of those people to be there. I wanted to be away from everyone, on my own . . . they said "don't push!" and that when I was so desperate to push, was such a battle—just *had* to when I got to that stage, just nothing else to do—and for some stupid lunatic to say 'hold it back!' It's a whole world you go back to, you know that from the beginning of time every person in that situation has got to push, you can feel it . . . I felt absolutely an animal, primitive . . . then I swore extremely violently, knocked the midwife's hat off and pushed . . . " (Valerie, speaking about her first born).

When modern births are conducted like an operation without an anesthetic, in which the patient is exposed to the callous matter of factness of surgeons removing the ripe appendage, the parturient's fears of her own death, separation, damage, and disclosure are largely ignored. Concern over the baby's ability to withstand labor and survive it intact, in short, to accomplish the transition almost replace earlier fears about the baby's normality, and can seriously hinder delivery. The woman may be convinced that the baby will not be born alive, or rather, that she cannot, will not be allowed to produce a real live baby. It is here that the midwife's role as surrogate mother becomes so important. The midwife's permission to have a baby, and encouragement to produce it, can positively affect the entire course of labor. The supreme maturational task of this third stage, before the delivery, involves preparation for her *active* role in labour and as a mother, (see Lampl de Groot, 1933) which will facilitate the exchange of fantasy baby for the real one met in childbirth. Thus, one might say the psychological tasks of these three stages involve *belief* first in the pregnancy, then in the fetus, and finally in the baby.

PREGNANCY AS A REHEARSAL

The stages the pregnant mother experiences in relation to her fetus are analogous to the stages Mahler (1975) postulates that a baby experiences in relation to its mother.

The early part of the first stage of pregnancy may be likened to Mahler's *"normal autistic phase,"* a state of "alert inactivity" during which the woman, like the newborn, is involved mainly in minimizing her disorientation and achieving a state of well-being without much recognition of its source. Later, the woman must accept the fetus as a unified part of herself. This is Mahler's *"symbiotic phase"* in which the "mother-child dual unity" are enveloped within a "common boundary." The difference is that in pregnancy, this is not a delusion but a reality. One woman described "a large magical bubble encapsulating (us) both and protecting us from danger and disease." This concept is similar to Mahler's "stimulus shield" (Mahler, 1975, p. 44).

The second stage of pregnancy is similar to that of "hatching" involving a gradual *"individuation"* of the fetus in the mother's mind, as well as "practice" separation through the tasks of "differentiation," "distancing," "boundary formation, and "disengagement." These culminate in the third stage of pregnancy with actual physical *separation* during birth and the *"rapprochement"* in the extrauterine reunion of mother and baby. The separation is greatly assisted, in pregnancy as in the mother–toddler relationship by the active role taken by the father (Mahler et al., 1975; Moore, 1968; Wisdom, 1976). Indeed, the presence of the husband in the delivery room may facilitate the birth-separation (Pines, verbal communication 1978b)

Thus, in my view, pregnancy may be regarded as a condensed rehearsal of the mother's future relationship with her baby in the 2 years following birth. Therefore, therapy and assistance during pregnancy have repercussions for parenthood far beyond a healthy "incubation" period.

PSYCHOTHERAPY WITH PREGNANT WOMEN

Psychotherapy aims to resolve earlier conflicts and deep-seated irrational emotions which interfere with everyday life and prevent the individual from achieving new maturational growth. Pregnancy is a time for reappraisal, redefinition, and potential psychic growth. It is a time of heightened sensitivity both to external events and internal sensations. It is a time of awakening of new emotions and a revival of forgotten feelings. It is a time for coming to terms with the past in order to better provide for a new and demanding future. Thus, the pregnant woman must undergo profound psychological and physical changes over a relatively short period of time, often necessitating some external therapeutic intervention to assist in her positive adaptation and completion of the maturational integrative tasks.

Individual Psychotherapy

The dramatic upsurge of emotions during pregnancy appears to transcend the usual boundary between what is allowed into conscious thought and what remains buried or inaccessible. Suddenly, the pregnant woman has immediate and direct access to her well of fantasies, her earlier modes of symbolic thinking, her awareness of secrets and intuitive understanding. She is "in touch" with her unconscious and at times feels almost overwhelmed by the power of the irrational within her. Paradoxically, pregnancy is a time of loneliness since she suddenly finds herself different from others, and unable to communicate the "mad" content of her experiences, which she recognizes and is embarrassed by. Her dreams, too, become extremely vivid, with often explicit symbolism and little attempt to "censor" or disguise forbidden content. In some ways psychotherapists may feel this situation resembles that of very neurotic, borderline, or even psychotic patients. However, there are several features of pregnant women that make psychotherapy with them unique:*

1. Their retention of almost intact ego resources despite the apparent disintegration of boundaries [somewhat similar to what has been observed with exceptionally creative people in therapy (Erikson, 1964; Heimann, 1977).] Also their powers of insight and interpretation of their own symbolism and primitive fantasies are at times remarkably astute.
2. Therapeutic intervention, clarification of the more cryptic messages or even just reassurance enabling the woman to examine her irrational feelings less fearfully achieve results reaching far beyond those normally achieved in therapy over a similar course of time. Women patients who become pregnant during an analysis also show an accelerated growth rate at this time (Pettitt, verbal communication, 1979).
3. Psychotherapy during pregnancy has a "built-in" termination date, and even if continued after the delivery, constitutes a different phase and situation. Therefore, pregnant women in therapy experience an urgency to

*These observations are based on work with individual patients who applied for treatment during pregnancy, and groups specifically formed for pregnant women.

achieve their growth and stability before the deadline of birth.

4. Thus, their own psychic growth and rebirth become symbolized by the growth of their pregnant bellies and the approaching birth of the child.

5. The "baby self" of the patient, often referred to in the abstract form with other patients in therapy, is very much present in her identification with the tangible baby within her womb.

6. The sanctity of the one-to-one relationship within individual treatment is "interrupted" at times by the actual presence of a third and sometimes a fourth person: the fetus, and in it, the representation of the sexual partner.

7. As pregnancy progresses, along with habituation to this situation, many of the strange experiences are assimilated and absorbed, and most are repressed and forgotten within weeks of giving birth.

8. In addition, unlike patients in analysis, there is no need for gradual build-up towards an interpretation of a delicate, deep, or powerful nature. The therapists may take chances and skip intermediate steps, get straight to the nitty gritty and, better still, receive immediate confirmation from the patient in the form of a hitherto forgotten memory, a sudden illumination, or a connecting spark.

Group Psychotherapy

Groups of pregnant women differ from most other psychotherapeutic groups in having all *female membership*. (Recently, with the advent of feminist therapeutic groups, this is becoming more common.) All group members may join the group together, or entry to the group may be staggered, however, unlike closed groups which begin and end together, each individual has her own termination date. Unlike "slow-open" (Foulkes,

1975) or open groups the termination date is built-in, i.e., determined by physical rather than psychological factors. Group members share a common life event in being pregnant, and all have sought help as a result of emotional difficulties during pregnancy. Also, in addition to the group members, there exist at least an equal number of "nonparticipant observers;" listening, responding, and recording namely, the fetuses. As a member of one of my groups remarked: "In analysis I could and did get away with lots unsaid or modified. Here I must be honest, otherwise the baby'll know that I'm lying or concealing things" (Helen.) Likewise, there are superstitions about the effect of verbalization on the fetus. ("Giving voice to my anger about the baby will hurt it.") Obviously these superstitions constitute one of the difficulties inherent in therapy with pregnant women.

Pregnancy itself is a period of *reticence.* There is a fear of diminishing the immediacy of the experience by analyzing or communicating intimate emotions; a fear of envoking the hand of fate or the evil-eye; and a reluctance to reveal the "bizarre" nature of her thoughts to nonpregnant listeners. This factor, plus the nonverbal nature of communication between mother and fetus, and the indefinable shared processes common to all pregnant women, mean that what is spelled out in the group is often for the leader's benefit, rather than for self-expression or group approval.

A typical feature of pregnancy is the absorption of earlier ideas and fantasies once the tasks of that phase are completed. After the birth there is complete and massive repression (Caplan, 1959) and restoral of defenses occurs. Thus, the group offers an ongoing "reminder" of forgotten experiences to those in later stages of pregnancy, and a record of "prehistoric times" once the baby is born. It also offers a "mutiple time-lapse view" of the rapidly changing state of equilibrium during pregnancy and its transitions. Both features, the reluctance of pregnant women to share their thoughts with nonpregnant outsiders and the later repression of the more fantastic of these, have contributed to the dearth of information about this state, and both are counteracted in the group setting, the group thereby offering a unique and rich potential for investigation and research.

FEATURES OF GROUP DYNAMICS AND TRANSFERENCE PHENOMENA IN PSYCHOTHERAPY GROUPS FOR PREGNANT WOMEN. The small, unstructured therapy group appears to develop according to a predictable format. Most writers agree that groups evolve from a regressed, undifferentiated primitive organization towards internal differentiation and maturity (Scheidlinger, 1968). This, of course, is also analogous to the developmental processes of the fetus within the womb, and hence has particular significance in groups of pregnant women. Saravay (1978) reviewing the literature on the small unstructured therapy group, proposes that in its evolution it recapitulates the stages of infantile development, beginning with regression to the oral dependent phase.

During group formation, the members of the group become dependent upon the leader. The leader represents the mother of the first half-year of life (Saravay, 1975; Scheidlinger, 1974). The group wish is to "achieve union" with the nourishing mother-leader (Anthony, 1967; Scheidlinger, 1968) and try to draw the leader into "the body of the group, attempting to erase the therapeutic barrier between them" (Saravay, 1978, p. 488). The mother is the symbol of "a unity which was disrupted by birth, by expulsion from the womb into the world" (Schindler, 1966. p. 201). The group itself comes to symbolize the *mother* (Schilder, 1940) *her body* (Saravay, 1975), *breast* (Bion, 1961; Schindler, 1966), and *the womb* (Schindler, 1966). Concurrently, there is a shift towards "empathic intuitive responses and primary processes" (Anthony, 1967). In the "pregnancy group" situation, these processes appear to be heightened. Regression, passivity, and dependence have already occurred in the individual as normal phenomena of pregnancy.

Further, an all-female group with a female leader is by virtue of the pregnancies already intensely preoccupied with motherhood, nourishing and being nourished, containing and merging. Orality is particularly emphasized by those in the first stage of pregnancy who are experiencing physical symptoms such as nausea, vomiting, food cravings, and hypersalivation. Saravay (1978) describes the oral-aggressive phase of group development in which members, enraged at the leader's neutral passivity, silence, and frustration of their wishes to be fed, begin to castigate themselves for their own silence and scapegoat silent members in their midst. "The members alternatively attack and support the scapegoat like a transitional object that contains parts of the self and the object" (p. 491). In the "pregnancy group," the leader is seen not only as the frustrating early mother, but is likened to the silent and inactive fetus, who becomes an additional scapegoat and transitional object.

Saravay (1978) further describes the anal retentive and anal expulsive maturational phases of the group. The former is characterized by ambivalence between the wish to maintain the dependent attachment to the leader and the wish to become independent, coupled with the rage at discovering that the fantasy of "blissful omnipotent duality" is at an end. The group wishes to dominate, control, and expel the leader and fear his "retaliatory elimination" of them (p. 493).

During the anal retentive phase, the members become a group with internalized norms and values, a cohesive sense of identity, and stabilized group boundaries. They consolidate their identities as individuals "distinct and separate although belonging to the group" (Saravay, 1978, p. 495). The leader is now seen as "a stabilized, positive, internalized object" (p. 494) while authority figures outside the group are invested with the hated qualities of the leader. "Independent decisions and initiative seem increasingly forbidden in the minds of the members" (p. 495) and the members yearn for a "Messiah" and have fantasies of an idealized "bisexual hero" (p. 495). In the "pregnancy group," once again these processes are evident, but have overdetermined connotations in that both these phases have their equivalents in the development of each pregnant woman's relationship with her fetus. With the quickening, her increased awareness of the baby as a separate loved/hated person contained within her leads to a preoccupation with the retention of the fetus and its expulsion in labor. In pregnancy groups, the leader at times represents the fetus to be expelled and the group represents the mother-in-labor. External authorities, particularly hospital or antenatal clinic health care workers, nurses, and midwives represent the early "enemy"—the abandoning, uncaring, bossy, envious mother who will rob the pregnant woman of her autonomy during childbirth, of the baby in the hospital, and of her feeding rights and decision-making capacity.

Saravay continues his account of group development with the phallic phase in which "Oedipal triangular relationships replace the earlier dyadic form" (Anthony, 1967) and the leader, previously seen as the preoedipal mother now represents the oedipal mother or father (Durkin, 1964). Much curiosity is displayed about the leader's private life, and frustration of this wish for intimacy symbolizes exclusion from the parental primal scene (p. 497). The concluding phase is that of the genital phase during which the healthier and more competent members of the group assume leadership, and the leader is viewed more realistically. "The threat of the dissolution of the group is met with fantasies of pregnancy and childbirth" (Slater, 1966; p. 499). In the "pregnancy group," these phases parallel the work done in the third stage of pregnancy in preparation for the triadic relationship that will include the baby, and the assumption of greater adult responsibilities, in view of the more realistic appraisal of the expectant mother's own mother, and concept of "motherliness." Each individual member has to prepare for her own labor as her delivery date approaches and the group participates in this process of separation. The group thus becomes the pregnant mother giving birth to her full-term fledgling; it is also the new mother identifying with and taking over from her own mother, i.e., the leader. At times, the leader is seen as the protective and caring father and the group as mother. The corporate fetuses become the child. As delivery approaches hospital authorities and particularly male doctors may be seen as omnipotent yet detached fathers, taking over when mother fails, "raping" (internal examinations), removing the baby by force (cesarean sections) and "castrating" (episiotomy). Needless to say, these cruel fathers have their kind and caring counterparts: "taking away the pain," "giving her a baby," "keeping the baby healthy." At such times, the leader may be seen as the well-meaning, but weak mother, the jealous mother, or eventually the helping, caring father's partner (like the midwife or nurse).It is noteworthy, that in the pregnancy group, it is the leader who at times is seen as the sexually inquisitive child excluded from the primal scene and curious about the contents of the pregnant bellies of the sexually knowledgable mothers.

VARIATIONS IN THE COUNTERTRANSFERENCE.   The countertransference is different when the therapist of a pregnant woman is pregnant herself and when she is not.

As a nonpregnant analyst working with pregnant women, I must always be aware of the possibility of my own envy being aroused while confronted with the patient's pregnancy. Forgotten and repressed elements from my own previous pregnancies are at times rearoused or evoked by the patient's experiences, accompanied by the attendant reactions of sympathy, empathy, and protectiveness towards the patient. I become, in some ways, pregnant with the expanding patient, nourishing her with transfusions distilled perhaps during my own pregnancies. At all times, I am aware of the *dual nature* of the countertransference. I have two clients, the mother and her fetus, and I alternate in my feelings on behalf of one or the other. In my interpretations, I find I have to achieve a fine balance between elucidating the pathologic while preserving those elements of idealization and fantasy that are necessary for the future welfare of the baby and mother. Thus, every mother must remain under the impression that her baby is best. It is by virtue of this capacity for idealization and a narcissistic identification with her baby and her own benevolent and somewhat altruistic mother that she will manage to achieve those impossible, never-ending feats required of a mother of a young infant. Winnicott (1956) has referred to this ability as "primary maternal preoccupation," a state of heightened sensitivity which develops towards the end of pregnancy and continues for a few weeks after the birth, following which it becomes repressed. He likens it to an illness "in which some aspect of the personality takes over temporarily" necessitating a "preoccupation with their own infant to the exclusion of other interests" (p. 302).

The second situation is when the analyst is pregnant and treating pregnant patients. At such times, in addition to my two clients (woman and her future baby) I have a third: my own fetus and the emotions it arouses in me. I am also aware of the additional time pressure (not only my patients deadline, but my own) and that the birth of my baby will mean a temporary cessation in my role as therapist and investigator. My own heightened emotional sensitivity can be an asset, an articulated tool in the therapy, however, I must be aware of its subjective edge, that is, what is aroused in me by virtue of my own pregnancy as opposed to a reflection of the patient's. I am aware of my own increased vulnerability to the patient's transference responses, especially her curiousity aroused by my "loss of neutrality." There also are my own "nesting" pressures, the impinging desire to remove my attention from the outside world and contemplate my own "innards."

Transference Reactions to the Pregnant Analyst Therapist

Analysis and psychoanalytically oriented therapies attempt to provide the patient with a "neutral" setting, offering opportunity for projecting his past emotional conflicts into the present situation. This neutrality is inevitably interfered with when the analyst becomes obviously pregnant. Many patients indicate that they have unconscious knowledge of the analyst's pregnancy even before it becomes visibly apparent and early experiences of maternal pregnancies are revived and often reenacted in the therapeutic setting. Lax (1969) has found that borderline patients are aware of the analyst's pregnancy sooner, have more intense reactions, and act out their conflicts more than neurotic patients. In the individual setting with nonpregnant patients, I have found as has Breen (1977) that my pregnancy aroused anger at the intrusion into the one-to-one relationship, envy of the fetus and my creative abilities, feelings of exclusion, and deprivation. With pregnant individual patients, few if any of these themes arose. The central issues were sibling rivalry, bewilderment at the "generational confusion" ("Grandmothers shouldn't have babies!") and concern that her infantile demands on me might damage, deprive, or anger my fetus. In mixed therapeutic groups, my experience has again been similar to Breen's. Sexual curiosity and accusations of sexual transgression and themes related to parental sexuality were common. I also found that the male patients, alarmed by the revival of their infantile wishes to bear a child, and the fear of the "potent, sexual woman," reacted with a "flight" into homosexual themes and interests. The females, identifying with me and excited by my procreativity, contemplated their own permitted or forbidden urges to propagate. In the "pregnancy group," however, what changed in the transference with the realization of my pregnancy, was the nature of the communication: I was no longer entitled to special asides, translations or interpretations of cryptic material, but was expected to "tune into the uterine waves."

CONCLUSION

The pregnant woman is in touch with primitive and unconscious forces which at times threaten to overwhelm her. Therapy at this time can help her to regain the equilibrium and achieve the maturational growth necessary for an enjoyable and healthy relationship with her child-to-be. The psychotherapist needs to provide a substitute for the network of social support that is no longer available to the pregnant woman in western society but also, is able to offer her special expertise. This kind of therapy offers an exciting and rewarding challenge to the therapist and a condensed learning experience unlike any other.

REFERENCES

Abraham, K. The female castration complex. (1920) In *Selected papers of Karl Abraham on psycho-analysis.* The International Psycho-Analytical Library, No. 13. London: Hogarth Press, 1949, pp. 338–369.

Abraham, K. An infantile theory of the origin of the female sex. (1923) In *Selected papers of Karl Abraham on psycho-analysis.* The International Psycho-Analytical Library, No. 13. London: Hogarth Press, 1949, p. 333.

Anthony, E. J. The generic elements in dyadic and group psychotherapy. *International Journal of Group Psychotherapy,* 1967, *17,* 57–70.

Balint, E. Technical problems found in the analysis of women by a woman analyst. *Bulletin of the British Psycho-Analytic Society,* 1972, *59,* 1–9.

Benedek, T. The organization of the reproductive drive. *International Journal of Psychoanalysis,* 1960, *41,* 1–15.

Benedek, T. The psychobiology of pregnancy. In E. J. Anthony & T. Benedek (Eds.), *Parenthood-Its psychology and psychopathology.* Boston: Little, Brown, 1970.

Benedek, T. Ambivalence, passion and love. *Journal of the American Psychoanalytic Associations,* 1977, *25*(1), 53–80.

Bibring, G. L. Some considerations of the psychological processes in pregnancy. *Psychoanalytic Study of the Child,* 1959, *14,* 113–121.

Bibring, G. L. Dwyer T. F., Huntington D. S., & Valenstein A. F. A Study of the psychological processes in pregnancy and of the earliest mother-child relationship. *Psychoanalytic Study of the Child,* 1961, *16,* 9–72.

Breen, D. *The birth of a first child.* London: Tavistock, 1975.

Caplan, G. *Concepts of mental health and consultation.* Washington, D.C.: U.S. Dept. of Health, Educational Welfare, Children's Bureau, 1959.

Davids, A., De Vault, S., & Talmadge, M. Psychological study of emotional factors in pregnancy: A preliminary report. *Psychosomatic Medicine,* 1961, *23* (2), 93–103.

Deutsch, H. *The psychology of women, Vol. 2. Motherhood.* London: Research Books, 1947.

Douglas, M. *Natural symbols.* London: Penguin Books, 1973.

Erikson, E. H. Inner and outer space; reflections on womanhood. *Daedalus,* 1964, *93*(2), 582–606.

Erikson, E. H. *Childhood and Society.* London: Penguin Books, 1965.

Freud, S. On the sexual theories of children, Vol. IX. *In The complete psychological works of Sigmund Freud,* London: Hogarth Press, 1908, pp. 205–226.

Greenberg, N. H., Loesch J. G., & Lakin M. Life situations associated with onset of pregnancy. *Psychosomatic Medicine,* 1959, *21*(4), 296–310.

Hanford, J. M. Pregnancy as a state of conflict. *Psychological Reports,* 1968, *22,* 1313–1342.

Hayman, A. Some aspects of regression in non-psychotic puerperal breakdown. *British Journal of Medical Psychology,* 1962, *35,* 135–145.

Heimann, P. Further observations on the analyst's cognitive processes. *Journal of the American Psychoanalytic Association,* 1977, *25*(2), 313–333.

Jacobson, E. On the development of the girl's wish for a child (1936). *Psychoanalytic Quarterly,* 1968, *37,* 523–538.

Jaffe, D. S. The masculine envy of woman's procreative function. *Journal of the American Psychoanalytic Association,* 1968, *16*(3), 521–548.

James, W. H. The effect of maternal psychological stress on the fetus. *British Journal of Psychiatry,* 1969, *115,* 811–825.

Jarrahi-Zadeh, A., Kane F. J. Jr., Van De Castle R. L., Lachenbruch P. A., & Ewing J. A., Emotional and cognitive changes in pregnancy and early puerperium. *British Journal of Psychiatry,* 1969, *115,* 797–806.

Kesternberg, J. S. Outside and inside, male and female. *Journal of the American Psychoanalytic Association,* 1968, *16*(3), 457–520.

Klein, H. R., Potter, H. W., & Dyk, R. B. *Anxiety in pregnancy and childbirth.* New York: Hoeber, 1950.

Klein, M. *The psychoanalysis of children.* New York: Norton, 1932.

Kumar, R., & Robson, K. Preliminary communication. Previous induced abortion and ante-natal depression in primaparae. *Psychology and Medicine,* 1978, *8,* 711–715.

Lampl de Groot, J. Problems of femininity. *Psychoanalytic Quarterly,* 1933, *2,* 489–518.

Lax, R. Some considerations of transference and countertransference manifestations evoked by the analyst's pregnancy. *International Journal of Psychoanalysis,* 1969, *50,* 363–372.

Lomas, P. Dread of envy as an aetiological factor in puerperal breakdown. *British Journal of Medical Psychology,* 1960, *33,* 105–112.

Mahler, M. S., Pine F., Bergman A. *The psychological birth of the human infant symbiosis and individuation.* London: Hutchinson, 1975.

Malinowski, B. *Magic, science and religion.* New York: Doubleday, 1955.

Menninger, W. C. The emotional factors in pregnancy. *Bulletin Menninger Clinic,* 1943, *7,* 15–24.

Pettitt, V. Personal communication, meeting of independent group of psychoanalysts. British Psychoanalytical Society, 1979, London.

Pines, D. Pregnancy and motherhood: Interaction between fantasy and reality. *British Journal of Medical Psychology,* 1972, *45,* 333–342.

Pines, D. On becoming a parent. *Journal of Child Psychotherapy,* 1978, *4*(4), 19–31.

Pines, D. Personal communication, Scientific Meeting. British Psychoanalytical Society, London, 1978b.

Rapoport, R. Normal crises: Family structure and mental health. *Family Practice,* 1963, *2,* 68–80.

Rosner, S. Further contributions to the psychic significance of the umbilicus. *International Review of Psychoanalysis,* 1978, *5*(1). 61–64.

Saravay, S. M. Group psychology and the structural theory: A revised psycho-analytical model of group psychology. *Journal of the American Psychoanalytic Association,* 1975, *23,* 69–89.

Saravay, S. M. A. Psychoanalytic theory of group development. *International Journal of Group Psychotherapy,* 1978, *28*(4), 481–505.

Scheidlinger, S. Group psychotherapy in the sixties. *American Journal of Psychotherapy,* 1968, *22,* 170–184.

Slater, P. E. *Microcosm: Structural, psychological and religious evolution in groups.* New York: Wiley, 1966.

Wenner, N. K., Cohen M. B., Weigart E. W., Kvarnes R. G., Ohaneson E. M., Fearing, J. M. Emotional problems in pregnancy. *Psychiatry,* 1969, *32*(4), 389–410.

Winnicott, D. W. The observation of infants in a set situation (1941), In D. W. Winnicott, *Collected papers.* London: Tavistock, 1958, pp. 33–51.

Winnicott, D. W. Primary maternal preoccupations (1956). In D. W. Winnicott, *Collected papers.* London: Tavistock, 1958, pp. 33–51.

Wisdom, J. O. The role of the father in the mind of the parents in psychoanalytic theory and in the life of the infant. *International Review of Psychoanalysis* 1976, *3*(2), 231–240.

BIBLIOGRAPHY

Bion, W. R. *Experiences in groups.* London: Tavistock, 1961.

Breen, D. Some differences between group and individual therapy in connection with the therapist's pregnancy. *International Journal of Group Psychotherapy,* 1977, *27*(4), 499–506.

Chasseguet-Smirgel, J. Freud and female sexuality. *International Journal of Psychoanalysis,* 1976, *57*(3), 275–286.

Chertok, L. *Motherhood and personality.* London: Tavistock, 1969.

Deutsch, H. The psychology of woman in relation to the functions of reproduction (1925). In R. Fliess (Ed.), *The psycho-analytic reader.* The International Psycho-Analytical Library, No. 38, London: Hogarth Press, 1950, pp. 165–180.

Durkin, H. *The group in depth.* New York: International Universities Press, 1964. Cited by S. M. Saravay: A psychoanalytic theory of group development. *International Journal of Group Psychotherapy,* 1978, *28*(4), 497.

Fast, I. Developments in gender identity: The original matrix. *International Review of Psychoanalysis,* 1978, *5*(3), 265–274.

Foulkes, S. H. *Group analytic psychotherapy—method and principles.* London, Gordon & Breach, 1975.

Freud, S. On transformation of instinct as exemplified by anal erotism, Vol. XVII. *The complete psychological works of Sigmund Freud.* London: Hogarth Press, 1917, pp. 125–134.

Freud, S. Some psychological consequences of anatomical distinction between the sexes. *The complete psychological works of Sigmund Freud,* Vol. XIX. London: Hogarth Press, 1925, pp. 243–260.

Gillespie, W. H. Woman and her discontents. *International Review Psychoanalysis* 1975, *2*(1), 1–10.

Horney, K. The denial of the vagina. *International Journal of Psychoanalysis,* 1933, *14,* 57–70.

Lewis, E. The management of stillbirth, Coping with an unreality. *Lancet,* 1976, *2,* 619–620.

Moore, R. E. Psychoanalytical reflections on the implications of recent physiological studies of the female orgasm. *Journal of the American Psychoanalytic Association,* 1968, *16,* 569–587.

Moore, B. E. Freud and female sexuality, A current view. *International Journal of Psychoanalysis* 1969, *57*(3), 287–300.

Pinney, E. L. Jr., Paul Schilder and group psychotherapy. The development of psychoanalytic group psychotherapy. *Psychiatric Quarterly,* 1978, *50*(2), 133–143.

Scheidlinger, S. On the concept of the "mother group." *International Journal of Psychotherapy,* 1974, *24,* 417–428.

Schindler, W. The role of the mother in group psychotherapy. *International Journal of Group Psychotherapy,* 1966, *16,* 198–202.

chapter 11

PSYCHOSEXUAL CONFLICTS IN EXPECTANT FATHERS

Sue Rosenberg Zalk

Men can not, and do not, become "parents" overnight. If one were to judge from the professional and social attention given to them, however, one might erroneously conclude otherwise. Expectant fathers in our society lack a group identity. Their needs and roles have traditionally been undefined. The transition from someone's son to someone's father is one of the major developmental tasks a man confronts. The issues and conflicts uncovered may reappear with each successive child; yet, the expectant father often goes ignored.

A pregnant woman, of course, goes through a shift and expansion in her identity. The changes she goes through during pregnancy and her sensitivity to the crises of her own childhood have been appreciated as necessary preparation for motherhood. It has been viewed as another developmental step for her. Similarly, a man does not become a psychological father with the birth of this child. The issues surrounding fatherhood and his evolving identity must begin long before the delivery date. Pregnancy, then, is a preparation period for men, also. It is a

9-month adapting period in which a man, like a woman, readies himself for parenthood.

How does a man prepare for parenthood? The expectant father confronts, once more, those developmental conflicts and conquests that were experienced as a child. The prospect of going from son to father, the thought of being *the* father in a family, the shifting roles and responsibilities, the increased dependency of others, marriage to a mother, the changing elements in his marriage, and then all this attention to childhood, inevitably triggers in all expectant fathers the surfacing of those psychosexual issues that were confronted in childhood. The expectant father experiences a rekindling of past issues of passivity and dependence, of separation, of aggression and sadomasochistic fantasies, and, of course, of oedipal dynamics.

Childhood dynamics are central elements in the adjustment to parenthood. It may be useful, therefore, to view the reemerging of psychosexual conflicts in expectant fathers as a developmental step in itself. It is a chance to rework some of those issues in order to ease the transition to the new role and identity. Dealing directly with the issues around parenthood seems to be easier for expectant mothers. Books have been written for and about her, and the pregnancy is something she cannot avoid. Men do not have these supports or signals, and at a time when they may be feeling very small themselves, they are told that their role is to "take care of the 'little woman' " (who is usually not looking very little). And although expectant fathers do dream more and fantasize more (Bittman & Zalk, 1978), they do so with less conscious awareness. Expectant fathers think more about their fathers and their childhood. They spend more time with their mothers, and take a keener interest in the events of her pregnancies (Bittman & Zalk, 1978; Colman & Colman, 1971; Liebenberg, 1969).

It is difficult to look at a child and not think about having been one. At the prospect of having one, the expectant father experiences, in the coming child, the events of his own childhood. But the expectations set for him (and the role he is expected to play is astonishingly undefined) offer him little direction or support for using these memories. He feels like he is floating around, bombarded with thoughts, fears, and fantasies. While the pregnant woman may be quick to connect emotional swings and concerns to the pregnancy, expectant fathers often show a range of bizarre behaviors and overt anxiety reactions, while dogmatically denying that it has anything at all to do with the pregnancy.

With unresolved conflicts reemerging, and defenses less effective, pregnancy can be a most stressful time for expectant fathers. A look at some examples of men's reactions to pregnancy and then a review of the emerging psychosexual conflicts that underlie them are necessary.

STRESS REACTIONS IN EXPECTANT FATHERS

Mr. A. verbalized ambivalence about fathering prior to the pregnancy. When his wife became pregnant, he expressed positive feelings about it. The one obvious noticeable change was a range of physical problems which began when the pregnancy was confirmed and ended "miraculously" after the birth. These physical difficulties included backaches, nausea (which diminished as the pregnancy progressed), gastrointestinal complaints, leg cramps, fatigue, and weight gain. All were symptoms associated with pregnancy.

Mr. B. had his first homosexual relationship when his wife became pregnant. He continued to have homosexual relationships (only occasionally having sex with his wife) throughout the remainder of the marriage, which lasted about 1 year after the birth of the child. As of writing this he was still an active homosexual.

Ms. C., an acquaintance, who heard I was doing research on expectant fathers, called to tell me that when she became pregnant her husband became enuretic. She asked if I wanted to interview her, since her husband was not available, he left about 6 months after the birth. Aside from the enuresis, which continued throughout the pregnancy, she reported that her husband had become impotent with her. She strongly suspected that he was having extramarital relationships, but I have no data on that.

Mr. D. felt depressed when his wife became pregnant. His behavior towards her was oversolicitous, overconcerned, and overdevoted. His reactions were clearly exaggerated. He would call the obstetrician frequently to tell him things about the pregnancy, to "tattle-tale" on his wife. He was critical of anything she did that he thought was the least bit disruptive to the fetus. This man had repetitive dreams of scuba diving, in which he was floating around under water with a long tube connecting him to an oxygen supply on the surface. It is interesting to note that Curtis (1955) found many references to water (classical symbols for birth and pregnancy) as well as to common childhood conceptions of pregnancy (i.e., activities related to eating, urinating, and defecating) in the fantasies and stories of expectant fathers. Four months after the birth, Mr. D. remarked that his wife had just stopped nursing, and he was feeling noticeably sad about it. He said he did not understand why since it meant considerable more freedom for the two of them. He talked about how no longer having the breast was a major deprivation for his daughter. This man experienced it as a personal loss.

Mr. E. is a classic example of a man who deals with the anxieties around the pregnancy by denying its existence. He insisted that he was unaffected by the pregnancy, that it was no "big thing," and that it had not interfered with his life in any way. He dragged his wife (who rather passively complied) on shopping trips, social events, and so forth, with an increased fervor. He proclaimed that he did not expect that his life would be any different after the baby was born. He refused to talk about baby plans and in the 8th month insisted that they had plenty of time to purchase the basics for a newborn. When his wife was in her 9th month they went to the country for the weekend. He said that if she went into labor he would have no trouble getting back in time. She did indeed go into labor in the country. They were 4 hours from the hospital at which she intended to deliver.

Mr. F., an expectant father, had purchased 15 t-shirts with the word "coach" written on the chest. He wore little else for the last 5 months of the pregnancy. He was asking "How do I fit into all of this?" He was also saying, "Hey, take note of me, I *do* fit into all of this!"

I am going to continue by summarizing some of the patterns that may appear with expectant fathers.

Mr. A, who was suffering from a range of physical symptoms that are often associated with pregnancy, was exhibiting a not uncommon phenomenon referred to as the Couvade syndrome. This syndrome is named after a ritual practiced in a number of unrelated preindustrial societies in different areas of the world. The ritual *couvade* (derived from the French word "couver" which means to brood or to hatch) is a pretense of childbirth. Although there are a range of variations, basically the ritual entails a simulated childbirth by the man at the time his wife goes into labor. In some cultures, the father practices a postnatal dietetic custom, demonstrating the intimate relationship perceived between the father and the child (Trethowan & Conlon, 1965). Numerous explanations have been offered for the ritual. Some of the most common is that it ensures the child's legitimacy, or that it is an example of sympathetic magic (Malinowski, 1937). Related to this is the notion of omnipotence of thought and the idea that the vicarious suffering of the man will relieve the woman (Trethowan & Conlon, 1965). Reik (1931), offering a psychodynamic explanation, viewed the ritual couvade as evidence of the man's ambivalence towards his wife and child. With love and hate existing simultaneously, the expectant father takes to bed on the pretense of service as a decoy for evil spirits, when in reality he is protecting his wife, and later his child, from his own hostility. Evidence for identification with, and envy of, the expectant woman as the underlying dynamic of this ritual have been presented (Munroe & Munroe, 1971; Trethowan & Conlon, 1965).

The Couvade syndrome is psychologically analogous to the ritual. Trethowan (1968), who has studied this syndrome, defines it as physical symptoms occurring in expectant fathers that are of psychogenic origin and have some symbolic relationship to the pregnancy. Thus, they often involve alimentary disorders but other symptoms appear as well. It is interesting to note that Inman (1941) found an increase in styes and tarsal cysts in men who were either expectant fathers or were having fantasies about childbirth. The couvade symptoms usually appear about the 3rd month of the pregnancy, may ease up in the middle months, become more intense in the last trimester, and disappear after the birth. Expectant fathers often do not connect these symptoms to the pregnancy. Estimates of its occurrence range from 9 percent to over one in three expectant fathers, depending upon the definition used (Trethowan & Conlon, 1965). We will return to the psychosexual conflicts represented in this syndrome.

There is widespread concern among expectant fathers that the child will be stillborn or deformed. They worry that their wives will die in childbirth or be badly mutilated by it. The expectant father may worry excessively and irrationally. Underlying these fears one often uncovers tremendous ambivalence toward the child and wife. Aggressive feelings towards the baby and/or wife are expressed as the fear that they will be hurt. One sees an extension of this in the often heard statement "I know it is irrational but I am afraid that if we have sexual intercourse it will hurt the child." This sentiment is expressed more frequently after the first trimester, which is the high-risk period for a woman prone to miscarry. The fear becomes more intense when the pregnancy "shows" and the movements of the fetus can be felt. The association between sex and aggression has long been recognized. An act that might otherwise be considered loving and giving, is instead seen as destructive. Unconscious hostility is defended against. Actually, a man might see the pregnancy as a result of an aggressive act. If his wife is having a difficult or uncomfortable pregnancy, this will, of course, intensify. The resulting guilt may have many expressions; depressive reactions are likely. The expectant father may be oversolicitious, may withdraw, or may deny the pregnancy. The association between sex and aggression can be found in the reactions some men have at the prospect of seeing their wives go through labor and delivery (Lacoursiere, 1972). It is difficult enough watching someone cared for in pain. If there is an overlay of sadistic feelings the prospect of the wife in pain will elicit tremendous anxiety. It is, after all, his "fault." (Although we can not go into it here, this is an important consideration when addressing the issues around a man's participation in the birthing.)

Related to the above issues is the excessive fear some expectant fathers have that *they* will die. That would certainly be an expedient way of avoiding the present and future situation. Every life insurance salesperson knows that an expectant father is a likely sale. Although this may be good planning on the part of the expectant father, the obsessiveness of the fear reveals the anger and hostility taking this defensive form.

Depression, denial, withdrawal, or exaggerated attentiveness may be camouflaging hostility. Little probing is needed, however, to see the aggressive expression in the act of "wife beating." Many battered women are first struck by their husbands when they become pregnant. Physical abuse directed at the pregnant women is much more frequent with unwanted pregnancies. Not uncommonly, the blows are directed towards the stomach. This is not only physical abuse directed towards the wife but it can be considered prenatal child abuse as well. The success of this method in eliminating this unborn competitor and upcoming responsibility through miscarriages can only be guessed at. It is frequently an indicator of future child abuse, and the precipitating stresses are numerous (Gelles, 1975).

Expectant fathers often experience a decreased sex drive (at least in relationship to their wives). They may, simultaneously, experience an increase in sexual fantasies about other women or men. Much has been written about the frequency in sexual activity of expectant couples. It has been, for the most part, seen as a function of the changes in the woman's mood and body. My own research revealed that men's sexual interest fluctuates in reaction to the pregnancy. Although many men find pregnant women a "turn-on," experience this time as a sexually heightened period and engage in sex with increased fervor, most men find themselves less interested in having sexual relations with their wives during the pregnancy. This lack of interest progresses with the pregnancy (Bittman & Zalk, 1978).

How do men explain their lack of libido? In addition to the expressed fears about hurting the fetus and/or wife, one hears things like, "It's just not a turn-on, pregnant women seem so asexual"; "it just doesn't seem right, sort of dirty"; "the fetus always gets active afterwards and I feel like I disrupted it, besides it always makes me feel like the baby has taken up my space inside my wife"; "her genitals are so full and swollen and wet and she seems so arousable, I feel like I could never match up, never satisfy her"; and, "the proximity to the fetus scares me. I know it is crazy but I feel like the fetus is going to hurt me. Reach down and grab my penis or bite it or something."

Sexual behavior becomes a likely activity ground for acting-out conflicts. Hartman and Nicolay (1966) compared a group of expectant fathers who had been arrested with a matched group of arrested men who were not expectant fathers. They found a significantly larger number of sexual crimes among expectant fathers. Among others, these included exhibitionism, pedophilia, rape or attempted rape, and lewd phone calls. They interpreted these behaviors as regressive adjustment reactions to anxiety about masculinity.

Other behaviors may serve to mask a depressive reaction and represent attempts to reduce anxiety. Some expectant fathers become reckless and impulsive. These men are more likely to get into trouble and to be accident prone (Curtis, 1955).

UNDERLYING PSYCHOSEXUAL CONFLICTS

Typically, the male child first identifies with his mother, then his father. It is his task to integrate these two roles. During a pregnancy, conflicts may arise and the expectant father revives and relives his identification with both his mother and his father in this particular developmental sequence (Benedek,

in a cross-cultural study, collected data on the ritual couvade and the Couvade syndrome. Their study included American men who were experiencing the couvade syndrome as well as expectant fathers who were without these symptoms. Two other cultures, one from British Honduras and one from western Kenya, were also studied. These investigators found that men exhibiting couvade symptoms or practicing the ritual were more likely to show more "masculinity" on overt measures (e.g., expressed attitudes, fighting) and more "femalelike" behaviors on covert measures (e.g., projective questions). They also found a higher incidence of father absences among American men demonstrating the syndrome and in cultures practicing the ritual. It is interesting to note that men suffering from the Couvade syndrome were more nurturing towards their newborns. In this we see one of the more positive outcomes of this identification.

Envy of the mother's ability to give birth has been documented many times (Boehm, 1939; Jacobson, 1960). It may find expression for the expectant father through competitiveness with his wife (van Leeuwen, 1966). Or, a man may attempt a kind of fusion with his wife, a merging of personalities, so that he can experience and control the pregnancy and birth (Liebenberg, 1969). Reaction formation is a common defense to this identification and envy. The expectant father may demonstrate exaggerated masculine behaviors, or he may have extramarital affairs. In this search for a masculine identity we see a preoedipal base for homosexual activities. Similarly, we can trace the compulsive regressive adjustment reactions of the expectant fathers who committed sexual crimes. In a more constructive light, some men take up hobbies, interests, and activities in an often successful attempt to be equally creative and productive (Boehm, 1930; Colman & Colman, 1971; van Leeuwen, 1966). If the pregnancy does not create too much anxiety, identification with the pregnant woman may assist a man in feeling empathy towards his wife, in involvement with the pregnancy and childcare, and in nurturing the child. All of which may provide gratification for the man.

Certainly, to some degree, men and women hope to recapture in marriage some of those lost moments with mother. This dependent relationship will be disrupted by the intruder-baby. Men whose dependency needs were insufficiently or ambivalently satisfied in childhood and whose choice of a wife was based primarily on these dependency needs will view the fetus as a rival for dependency (rather than as a phallic competitor as others have stressed) (Lacoursiere, 1972). Not infrequently, such dependent men marry controlling women, who do, indeed, see their husbands as their children. With the prospect of having her own "real" baby the feared rejection may, indeed, occur (Towne & Afterman, 1955). But even if the wife does not respond this way, the fear of loss of love and attention can be experienced intensely. The pregnancy becomes evidence that the expectant father is no longer a child, confronts him with his increased adult responsibilities, and results in the frustration of his dependency needs. The fetus, and later the newborn, will be assigned sibling status and viewed as a competitor. Jealousy and anger at the child and wife-mother for her betrayal may follow. This will be more intense for the expectant father who had younger siblings and did in reality experience a loss of attention and care as a result. Regressive behaviors and identification with the baby are not uncommon and are often found in dreams and fantasies, as well as behaviors of expectant fathers. The expectant father may project his own fantasies on to the child and attribute to the baby the same unacceptable feelings he had towards his father (Towne & Afterman, 1955).

These conflicts may reactivate earlier aggressive feelings towards family members. The expectant father will direct his aggressive feelings towards his wife and/or child and generally experience an accompanying guilt. It may take the form of depression, which may be masked by self-destructive behaviors, such as recklessness or accident proneness. Expectant fathers may show signs of insomnia, lack of concentration, impotence, and anxiety. The hostility may be directed out, as in physical aggression towards the wife or child. After the birth, this may be revealed in careless or neglectful handling of the child (Ginath, 1974). The expectant father may become unfaithful in a search for a new caretaker. He may even abandon his wife during the pregnancy or shortly thereafter (many couples show the seeds for divorce during the pregnancy). One may see evidence of these conflicts with the expectant father who is excessively solicitous and spoiling or who shows an exaggerated and unfounded concern about the possibility of damage happening to the wife or child during childbirth or love making.

Although it will be anxiety provoking, expectant fatherhood is not always quite this problematic, and it is easy to end this chapter on a positive note. Dependency and identity issues will inevitably resurface when a man is confronted with the prospect of becoming a father. They are a signal to the man that there are unresolved issues and things to attend to. If the anxiety is not too intense, they provide a man with a second chance to rework them, a necessary preparation for fatherhood. They stimulate the psychological processes required for a man to make that transition from "son to father." This is the task for this developmental stage of expectant fatherhood.

REFERENCES

Benedek, T. Parenthood as a developmental phase. *Journal of the American Psychoanalytic Association*, 1959, *7*, 389–417.

Bittman, S., & Zalk, S. R. *Expectant fathers.* New York: Hawthorn Books, 1978.

Boehm, F. The femininity complex in man. *International Journal of Psychoanalysis*, 1930, *11*, 444–469.

Colman, A. D., & Colman, L. *Pregnancy: the psychological experience.* New York: Seabury Press, 1971.

Curtis, J. A. A psychiatric study of 55 expectant fathers. *U.S. Armed Forces Medical Journal*, 1955, *6*, 937–950.

Freeman, T. Pregnancy as a precipitant of mental illness in men. *British Journal of Medical Psychology,* 1951, *24,* 49–54.

Gelles, P. Violence and pregnancy: A note on the extent of the problem and needed services. *Family Coordinator,* 1975, *24 (4),* 81–86.

Ginath, Y. Psychoses in males in relation to their wives pregnancy and childbirth. *Israel Annuals of Psychiatry and Related Disciplines,* 1974, *12,* 227–237.

Hartman, A., & Nicolay, R. Sexually deviant behavior in expectant fathers. *Journal of abnormal and social psychology,* 1966, *71,* 232–234.

Inman, W. S. The couvade in modern England. *British Journal of Medical Psychology,* 1941–43, *19,* 37–55.

Jacobson, E. Development of the wish for a child in boys. *Psychoanalytic Study of the Child,* 1950, *5,* 139–159.

Jarvis, W. Some effects of pregnancy and childbirth on men. *American Psychoanalytic Association Journal,* 1962, *10,* 689–700.

King, E. The pregnant father. *Bulletin of the American College of Nurses and Midwives,* 1968, *13,* 19–25.

Lacoursiere, R. A. Fatherhood and mental illness: a review and new material. *Psychiatric Quarterly,* 1972, *46,* 109–124.

Liebenberg, B. Expectant fathers. *Child and Family,* 1969, *8 (3),* 265–277.

Malinowsky, B. *Sex and repression in savage society.* London: Kegan Paul, 1937.

Munroe, R. L., & Munroe, R. H. Male pregnancy symptoms and cross-sex identity in three societies. *Journal of Social Psychology,* 1971, *84,* 11–25.

Reik, T. *Ritual: psychoanalytic studies,* 2nd ed. New York: Farrar, Straus, 1946.

Towne, R. D., & Afterman, J. Psychosis in males related to parenthood. *Bulletin of the Menninger Clinic,* 1955, *19,* 19–26.

Trethowan, W. H. The couvade syndrome—some further observations. *Journal of Psychosomatic Research,* 1968, *12,* 107–115.

Trethowan, W. H., & Conlon, M. F. The couvade syndrome. *British Journal of Psychiatry,* 1965, *111,* 57–66.

van Leeuwen, K. Pregnancy envy in the male. *International Journal of Psychoanalysis,* 1966, *47,* 319–324.

Wainwright, W. H. Fatherhood as a precipitant of mental illness. *American Journal of Psychiatry,* 1966, *123,* 40–44.

Zilboorg, G. Depressive reactions related to parenthood. *American Journal of Psychiatry,* 1931, *87,* 927–962.

chapter 12

THE PREGNANT FATHER

Harriet R. Barry
Stephen Paul Adler

Many expectant fathers report experiencing disappointments, frustrations, and feelings of being excluded or displaced during the prenatal period. In a time in social history when sexism and roles are frequently being discussed, it is of great and timely importance to articulate the father's experience during pregnancy and also to find ways to foster paternal bonding to child, mother, and the family unit. This chapter explores the father's experiences in unplanned (but not to be aborted) and in planned pregnancies. Using the traditional trimester division of pregnancy, a general outline of the normal psychological and psychosomatic reactions of the expectant father are represented. The role of the childbirth educator and of the psychotherapist in facilitating a fulfilling pregnancy experience for the father are discussed.

The observations and thinking for this paper are based on samples of middle-income white (60 percent), middle-income orthodox Jewish (25 percent), lower-income black (10 percent) and Hispanic (5 percent) populations attending childbirth education classes in Brooklyn, New York. The underrepresentation of the lower income groups—who make up a majority of clinic patients—is a result of their lack of information about childbirth education rather than their lack of interest. Until recently, Lamaze literature was available only in English and childbirth educators were limited in presenting material to non-English-speaking groups. Newly developed programs, such as those at Metropolitan Hospital, New York, and the Wholistic Childbirth Preparation and Family Center of New York have found that low-income Spanish-speaking students' interest and motivation in childbirth education is equal to that of any other socioeconomic group. Further, the need for support services for fathers in these groups is at least equal to the needs of middle-income and English-speaking fathers.

UNPLANNED PREGNANCIES

During the first trimester, the pregnant father's feelings are dependent, in part, upon whether or not the couple is married and the pregnancy is planned. In general, it is easier for married couples, who are more within the familial law structure, to work through and to accept unplanned pregnancies. Unmarried couples have additional conflicts to face if they accept the pregnancy: Should they marry or remain single? Is the child legitimate or illegitimate? What should they surname the baby?

The initial response of the father in cases of unplanned pregnancies is usually shock followed by disbelief. The expectant father may even deny that the child is his. It is not unusual for him to believe that the pregnancy was part of the woman's scheme to entrap him into a greater commitment to the relationship. Feelings of antagonism toward the woman, which he might have had prior to the pregnancy, may become magnified and contribute to his expressions of hostility. Also, the father may see the unborn child as a potential rival. As the pregnancy continues, growing negative feelings and self-pity can result in

increasing expressions of hostility toward the mother and unborn child. If the father's initial negative feelings are not adequately processed, a cycle is established leading the mother to
feel hostile toward and possibly reject both the father and the
unborn child. As the cycle continues, the father may end up
leaving the mother and the baby. In order to prevent the father
from leaving the relationship in a destructive way, this cycle
must be broken. If the father is aided in exploring his feelings
and attitudes, both stated and unstated, it is possible that he
may be able to leave the relationship or move in and out of the
relationship in a constructive rather than a destructive manner.
If the father can be aware of and be helped to understand and
to accept his changing responses and feelings, he might then
become the most significant support person for the pregnant
woman. Sensitive childbirth education classes and/or psychotherapeutic intervention can contribute to helping the man
understand and accept his feelings, responsibilities, and roles in
the pregnancy experience.

The father's presence at prenatal examination visits and at
prenatal education classes should be strongly encouraged by the
obstetrician/midwife. Although he might be resistant and/or
passive, his attendance is a symbolic statement that he is a part
of the pregnancy process, delivery, and labor. Also, his presence
symbolically establishes his wish to share the parenting role.

It is imperative that physicians and midwives recognize
that in involving the father prenatally, they are making an
important contribution to the facilitation or inhibition of the
father's communication and interaction in the family dyad/-
triad. The childbirth educator both supports the obstetric case
management and, via a group process involving other couples,
deals with anxieties and real and unreal expectations that need
to be confronted by prospective parents. Through understanding, the positive nature of the couple's relationships
(whether it is permanent or not is not the issue) can be enhanced
and the birth can be a more positive experience. Both the man
and the woman can experience and offer support. Many psy-

chological studies, (e.g., Deutscher, 1969) indicate that a constructive environment during pregnancy increases the child's chances for healthy development in his/her early years and the prognosis for the couple is in favor of a better family life.

The psychotherapist working with the father in the unplanned pregnancy should take an active, responsive, but not responsible role. This is not the time for long-term replaying of past history. In fact, the father's history only as it directly refers to and interferes with his making clear and fairly immediate decisions needs to be processed. The therapist must not fall into the trap of being the decision maker. The only other role the therapist should take is in supporting the father in his carrying out in a responsible manner any decisions he might make.

PLANNED PREGNANCIES

In most planned pregnancy experiences, the expectant father's feelings take a somewhat different course. Although some ambivalence, anxiety, or guilt are frequently apparent, the expectant father frequently reports that he feels masculine and powerful in his male image and more responsible, loving, and protective toward his mate.[1] He becomes aware and awakens to his lack of or accomplished professional and financial achievements. He is most often optimistic, cheerful, and anticipatory towards the birth of his child. Often it is the first time he becomes aware of his health and how he will financially provide for his family alive or dead.

These feelings are encouraged by his interactions with the pregnant woman. If she, however, is uncommitted or resentful to the planned pregnancy, and/or if her pregnancy results in a wish to punish the father ("I want him to see what I go through." "I want him to see how I suffer."), in many cases guilt may be his predominant feeling.

[1] Based on a survey of 1500 expectant fathers conducted by Harriet R. Barry from 1975 to 1979.

By the beginning of the second trimester (4th, 5th, 6th months), most couples have made the appropriate adjustments and commitments to the pregnancy. Sexual feelings and fulfillment usually reach greatest intensity during this period. Often this trimester offers an idyllic honeymoon phase. There is little, if any, change in life-style. The pregnant woman usually feels physically well. The expectant father may become more physically and psychically connected to the woman and the baby, and he may even experience symptoms of pregnancy: gastrointestinal upset, increased eating, weight gain, and extreme tiredness. The second trimester can offer a second chance opportunity to improve the quality of the couple's relationship.

The expectant father's feelings focus suddenly on the visible body change that occur in the woman. It is a most propitious time for the professional to help him understand his reactions to the woman's changing body. Her body changes can trigger guilt, shock, or disgust which, in turn, can lead to sexual impotency in the second and third trimesters as well as long-term effects. Social and cultural conditioning and misconceptions (e.g., intercourse will damage the unborn baby) can interfere with their sexual life. These misconceptions tend to lose their effectiveness in directing the father's sexual feelings and responses when they are discussed fully. Further, when the father's role as the most significant support person to the pregnant woman is discussed, guilt feelings and associated anxieties can be rechannelled into more productive behavior often leading to feelings of responsiveness and tenderness toward the woman.

The third trimester is a time of intense mood changes for most women as well as the depletion of physical stamina (influenced by hormonal changes, season, and profession). The pregnant father is emotionally and psychologically called upon to give a great deal. He is concerned for the mother's well-being and often becomes more protective. He takes over many of the physical chores. He becomes her main physical and psychological support. If the pregnant woman transfers her needs to the physician, the father may begin to feel quite unimportant and helpless, thus introducing a new conflict to the situation.

The father's anger and resentment may grow if he is made to feel powerless. He may be excluded from office visits and examinations. Physicians tend not to get involved in the couple's relationship and thus may not be aware of the importance of unifying and solidifying their needs for each other during this trimester. Excluding the father most frequently produces feelings of alienation and some distancing from the mother. It becomes paramount for the physician or midwife as well as other professionals to assess the appropriate degree of inclusion needed and wanted by each couple and to make a concerted effort to include the father.

Prenatal management during the third trimester often prescribes sexual abstinence for the couple. The psychotherapist needs to be aware of the aforementioned and be ready to offer alternatives leading to reduced sexual tension and the couple's mutual satisfaction. Accomplishing this involves open discussion of human sexuality and comfortable alternatives that need not be considered perversions or pornography. Bittman and Zalk (1978) discuss some sexual alternatives.

There are other preoccupations that occur at this time. The safety of the mother and baby during labor and delivery become an issue. The father worries about getting to the hospital on time; he fears that he will have to deliver the baby. It is extremely important that his concerns be treated with dignity, respect, and that he intelligently receive detailed explanations as to what is occurring. He must not have his father/husband/male image weakened in his own eyes or the eyes of his woman. His own self-esteem must be maintained for the immediate long-term relationship to his child and family.

There is no doubt that the childbirth preparation classes and ongoing psychotherapeutic support help the father understand and accept his emotional needs and rights and put family bonding and integration into a more constructive perspective. It is important that the counselor remember that during the pregnancy the father's past history and/or his images of his parents' relationship to him be explored only if brought up and pursued by the expectant father himself. If provoked before the birth of the child, these issues tend to increase anxiety and may interfere with the productive playing out of his pregnant parental role.

The authors' viewpoint is not meant to be a panacea in providing the answer to a healthy childbirth experience and future family life. If the role and feelings of the expectant father are not considered, however, the job of professionals working with pregnancy and childbirth is not complete. Perhaps it is time to consider birthing practices in relationship to human needs rather than efficient medical management. Although working with fathers takes additional time, effort, and expertise, knowledgable guidance can enhance the pregnancy and childbirth experience for all concerned.

REFERENCES

Bittman, S., & Zalk, S. *Expectant fathers.* New York: Hawthorne, 1978.
Deutscher, M. Brief family therapy in the course of the first pregnancy: A clinical note. *Contemporary Psychoanalysis,* 1969, *7,* 21–35.

chapter 13

ATTITUDES TOWARD THE PREGNANT BODY

Harriet R. Barry

Self-satisfaction with her body and body image is important for a woman to accept and to fully enjoy her pregnancy. Many factors including cultural and social norms, maternal age, whether the pregnancy is planned or unplanned, and attitudes toward her body prior to pregnancy affect a woman's adjustments and attitudes. This chapter considers some of these factors and how Lamaze or other childbirth education can foster development of a positive body image during pregnancy.

Body image develops and is influenced by the social and physical environment. Historically, attitudes toward the pregnant body have not always been favorable (Tanzer, 1972). In ancient Egypt, lying-in women were considered to be unclean and subject to purification and isolation. The Greeks banned birth in their temples (Canfrani, 1960), and any woman who did not make her pregnancy known was subject to punishment. In some cultures, attempts were made to hide the pregnant body by homemade garments or pregnant women stayed home once their "condition" was obvious.

In the United States, pregnancy and childbirth have achieved "illness status." In labor, for example, women are frequently restricted to bed and moved to a delivery table in a room which looks like and can serve as an operating room. During labor and delivery, women may be given drugs or anesthesias which may lead her to feel that her body was not able to perform normally or adequately. This might not only have physical effects; self-esteem also may suffer.

Fantasies that pregnancy will cause the woman's body to have sagging breasts, stretch marks, fatness, or a slackening vagina or that her sexual desires will decrease during and after pregnancy, may affect men and women's reactions to pregnant bodies. Fears that sexual intercourse will injure the unborn child may result in sexual abstinence and/or stifled physical contact. If these fantasies and attitudes are not discussed and clarified adequately, there may be negative affects on the woman's body image and self-esteem, and on the couple's sexual and emotional relationship.

Age also may affect how a woman responds to her pregnant body. An adolescent may find the body changes of pregnancy, compounded by the enormous normal body changes of puberty, to be overwhelming. Older women, may be concerned about the adequacy of their bodies to handle the stress. These and all women profit from concrete information about the nonpregnant and pregnant body, its functioning processes, needs, and signals.

A planned or unplanned pregnancy affects a woman's responses to her changing pregnant body. In fact, one of the greatest differences in planned and unplanned pregnancies is the degree of threat to body image and self-esteem. Compared to women with planned pregnancies, women with unplanned or ambivalent pregnancies are more likely to experience physical symptoms such as vomiting and dizziness during the first trimester, and to eat inadequately during the second trimester. Women with unplanned, ambivalent pregnancies may attempt to hide the pregnancy and maintain a slim or nonpregnant body image for as long as possible. They may interpret remarks regarding their appearance to mean that they are no longer as beautiful or as lovely as before. Women with planned pregnancies who had negative body images prior to the pregnancy, might buy and wear maternity clothes early to let others know that their new body changes reflect pregnancy.

Women with negative body images prior to pregnancy may experience difficult adjustments to their new bodies. To foster the development of a positive connection between mind and body, these pregnant women especially might be encouraged to attend antepartum exercise classes. The second trimester appears to be a most propitious time to involve women in tailored exercise or body therapy programs (Kitzinger, 1970). Hormonal production (e.g., relaxin) allows the woman, perhaps more than prior to pregnancy, to attain flexibility in the use of her body. Women have reported that programs such as the Alexander Technique result in feelings of well-being and sensory awareness that enhances their self-image. If specific exercise/classes for the pregnant woman are not available, other supports, such as groups and childbirth education classes, where the body changes are discussed openly will be crucial to develop and maintain a positive body image. Because the pregnant body is the first "nest" for the child, positive feelings toward her body may contribute to the woman's beliefs concerning her ability to develop and provide a future home.

Medical records, for the most part, do not hint at the physical stress she is experiencing, and its affect on self-concept. The vocabulary of women in the third trimester often reflects their very apparent body changes changes and self-images. "I will bear it in mind"; "full"; "refrigerator bursting"; "seed"; and "fruitful" are commonly used words and phrases. Her expanding world of hope, fear, and anticipation is reflected in the physical reality of her enlarging abdomen. As the pregnancy nears term, the woman's vocabulary begins to include phrases like "I feel like an elephant"; "house"; "watermelons"; "blimps." Her body/mind connection is further complicated by the fact that at the end of the pregnancy she may feel physically and emotionally assaulted. In the physicians office or hospital, the abdomen usually is draped or covered and the genital area is blocked from self-view while open to the view of the gynecologist or nurse. When the genital area, usually the last to be uncovered in sexual/sensual life experiences is closed to self and open to others, there may be negative self-body ramifications.

The skilled Lamaze instructor can positively influence the woman's body image. In the childbirth education group, there is a common shared experience of enlarged abdomens. A segment of the Lamaze preparation deals with the anatomy and physiology of pregnancy, labor, and delivery. Visual aids, common experiences, and open discussion help a woman to understand and to accept her body and its changes. The relaxation techniques, which allow both the woman alone and couple to work with her body, also help her to establish a more positive body image. The woman is guided through an experience of sensory awareness and is encouraged to verbalize what feels good and what she likes. She is encouraged to realize that she has choices in how she experiences her own body. The man is encouraged to participate in the work with the woman's body, thereby positively affecting his relationship to her, her body, and the unborn child. His acceptance of her body affects her own feelings of desirability.

The woman who has a positive body image during pregnancy and delivery is more likely to have a positive childbirth experience and transition to parenthood. Following delivery, her body image will reflect the many attitudes, sensations, and images she experienced during her pregnancy. If adequately processed, her reactions toward her body prior to and during pregnancy can contribute significantly to development of positive self-esteem which can affect positively her ability and desire to mother.

REFERENCES

Canfrani, T. *A short history of obstetrics and gynecology.* Springfield, Ill.: Charles C Thomas, 1960.

Jones, Frank Pierce. *Body awareness.* Schocken, N.Y., 1976.

Kitzinger, S. *The experience of childbirth.* New York: Penguin, 1970.

Moore, Dianne S. MN. CNM, Journal of Nurse Midwifery. Vol. 22, No. 4, Winter 1978.

Tanzer, D. *Why natural childbirth.* New York: Doubleday, 1969.

chapter 14

THE THERAPIST'S PREGNANCY

Laura Barbanel

A therapist's pregnancy *must* be dealt with in therapy. Avoiding the discussion of the therapist's pregnancy—whether or not the patient spontaneously brings it up—involves the denial of patient's perceptions. These perceptions properly belong in the treatment situation. Four clinical examples will be presented, two for whom the therapist's pregnancy led to greater integration and growth, and two for whom it resulted in greater disruption.

A subsidiary thesis relates to the topic of miscarriage, a topic even more absent in the psychological literature. Here too, to deny and to avoid the discussion of the topic where the therapist clearly has experienced a miscarriage is to deny the patient's experience and to avoid an opportunity for associations that can offer rich material for therapeutic exploration.

Having experienced four pregnancies in 5 years, two resulting in live births and two in miscarriages (one late enough in the pregnancy to necessitate sharing with patients the sad news), it became clear that the patient's reactions to the pregnancies was an important ingredient in their treatment. Some patients openly asked if I were pregnant; others symbolically (by dreams) announced recognition of my condition while others had to be told of my pregnancy. Among the issues that required consideration were transference and countertransferences aroused; relationship of the patient's dynamics to recognition of a therapist's pregnancy; and the issue of the therapist's pregnancy as related to the broader issue of the woman therapist.

Although there is some literature on the topic, it is scattered and incomplete. It is my contention that this is not accidental, but reflects certain notions about therapists, pregnancy, and the combination of the two. Lax (1969) cited only two previous papers on therapists' pregnancies (Hannett, 1949; Le Bow, 1963). In a more recent review of the literature, five more articles on the topic (Benedek, 1973; Browning, 1974; Nadelson et al., 1974; Paluzny & Poznanski, 1971; Schwartz, 1975), and one chapter in a book (Balsam, 1974) were found. Although these six articles do not constitute a complete treatment of the topic, the contrast between the period before 1969 and after is striking. The simplest explanation for this change might be an increase in female therapists of childbearing age who are seeing patients and having children. On the other hand, it may be related to social or psychological changes resulting in female therapists becoming more likely to write about their experiences with patients during their pregnancies. Statistics are not available to test either hypothesis, but I suspect the latter to be true. I believe that in the past there was denial of the therapist's pregnancy in the literature, by the therapist and by the patient. The recent openness of discussion is worthy of greater exploration.

Many factors support denial, by both the patient and the therapist. The topic of pregnancy is generally not discussed in our society. Many women avoid "telling" that they are pregnant until the pregnancy is quite advanced. It is not considered polite to ask a woman if she is pregnant. Historically, women went to great pains to hide their pregnancies. Among Orthodox Jewish women, for example, the fact that a woman is pregnant is not mentioned throughout her entire pregnancy. Euphemisms are used to describe pregnancy, e.g., "expecting," "in a family way," "with child." In the literature on pregnancy and its effects on the pregnant woman, there is a smattering of discussion of the taboo against discussing one's own pregnancy. Klein (with Potter and Dyk, 1950; Klein 1957) suggests that some of this taboo relates to the fears about pregnancy and the notion that talking about it might make the feared outcome come true. Childbirth is associated with pain, danger, and death. The pain of childbirth, the danger to the mother and child, have an enormous written and oral history. From biblical times onward, the fears and suffering of women have been associated with childbearing. From generation to generation, the stories, myths, and tragedies get passed on. The incidence of death in childbirth has been reduced enormously in our society, yet birth and death are clearly associated in the unconscious and sometimes conscious awareness of most people. Both birth and death are mysterious and unpredictable. Both resist human control and have elaborate mythologies, religious rituals, superstitions, and fears surrounding them.

In therapy, presumably, these taboos on discussion should not operate. In the therapeutic setting, the unthinkable and unmentionable can be thought and mentioned. Sexual associations, angry thoughts, even homicidal impulses, not mentioned in polite company, are all permitted in the therapeutic session. However, all of this is with the basic ground rule accepted by most therapists, that the therapist remain anonymous. The therapist's pregnancy is a most personal matter, involving a very blatant admission of sexual activity. It is a statement about a relationship to a man and to a family. Not only is the therapist's pregnancy clearly a violation of the rule of the therapist's keeping her personal life out of the consulting room, but it is a violation that is unique to women therapists. Pregnancy is certainly not part of the therapist-expert-doctor (i.e., male) role.

It is, therefore, out of the purview of that role. If to be female is somewhat suspect to the therapist's role, then to be pregnant is to be guilty. Guilty because one's female functions intrude and, paradoxically, because one cannot fulfill the female functioning of mothering one's patients. It follows from this that if the pregnancy has to occur, it is certainly better that it be kept out of the consulting room as much as possible.

If the therapist's pregnancy is not discussed, the patient and therapist can recreate the parent–child situation, where certain secrets, namely of the bedroom, are not discussed. As we know in relation to secrets that parents attempt to keep from their children, the children always "know" on some level. Child therapists help children to verbalize this knowledge. To not do so with adult patients, because of some notion about anonymity, would be carrying the notion of anonymity to an extreme which Stone (1961) describes as involving "pathologic or pathogenic avoidances" (p. 37).

Patients' "knowing" of the therapist's pregnancy can be expressed many ways. Often, this "knowing" is expressed quite early in the pregnancy. For example, a 26-year-old female patient noted the abstract design on my print dress, interrupted herself in the middle of a completely different topic, and exclaimed, "the design on your dress looks like fallopian tubes." This dress had been worn before with no comment from her. This comment was made on the exact day that my pregnancy had been verified. Around the same time in another pregnancy, an unmarried female patient reported neglecting birth control for the first time. Another patient became pregnant and had an abortion. A fourth patient began to report dreams about babies. It is certainly possible that these were coincidences, and were related to the transference relationship, independent of my pregnancy. However, it is not likely. It is more likely that these are instances of different levels of "knowing." Pregnancy is an area where the irrational abounds. Bibring (1959) writes that with the increasing emphasis on the "scientific" in our society, less attention is paid to the irrational, emotional aspects of human experience. Such instances, as described above, strike one as that irrational side of human understanding.

Assuming that each of the above examples indicates the patient's subliminal awareness of the therapist's pregnancy, this awareness might be regarded as a kind of primitive identification with the therapist and therefore with her pregnancy. This plausible explanation is difficult to prove. Of the four patients cited, not one of them was the kind of patient who somehow "guessed" or intuitively "knew" other things about the therapist's life. Rather, the receptiveness seemed related specifically to pregnancy and to childbirth and the meaning that it held for the patients. For each of the patients, the therapist's pregnancy caused a great deal of upheaval. It is possible that the most unrelated patients make the most primitive identifications, and notice the pregnancy the earliest. Lax (1969) found that her borderline patients became aware of her pregnancy much earlier, and reacted with greater intensity. Also, she noted that patients diagnosed as borderline found it much more difficult to differentiate between transference and reality aspects of the situation.

The amount of denial some patients use in relation to the pregnancy is enormous. Lax (1969) reported that male patients use denial to a much greater degree than do female patients. A 20-year-old male patient, whom I started to see during the 5th month of my first pregnancy, was told that I would be away for 8 weeks in the summer. I did not mention that I was pregnant. He persisted in not "noticing." When I did tell him, at a point where not noticing was quite unlikely, his reaction was "You mean you won't be traveling this summer?" Although it may be true, as Lax found, that for male patients the therapist's pregnancy causes less upheaval than for female patients, this was not the case for this young man. The extent of his upheaval will be described in case C.

Other denying patients notice some "change" but do not attribute it to pregnancy. Several patients commented on my gaining weight, and associated it to my overeating because of neurotic problems. In fantasizing about the kinds of problems I might have, the problem of not having a man and of being homosexual were mentioned frequently. When these patients were asked what else getting heavier might be associated with, two patients replied: "You're not pregnant!" In both cases, it was preferable for the therapist to be neurotic, without a man, and/or homosexual to her being pregnant. During one of my pregnancies, a patient noted that I had had my hair cut, but did not note the pregnancy. Along with her comment about my hair being cut (a rather minor change compared to the physical changes related to a 6-month pregnancy) she stated, "I never notice anything usually." Another patient said that my style of dress had changed in the last 6 months; she wondered why.

Denial or avoidance on the patient's part is easy for the pregnant therapist to reinforce due in part to countertransference issues. Some (e.g., Balsam, 1974; Paluzny & Poznanski, 1971) have noted the tendency of pregnant women to withdraw psychic energy from the outside world and to retreat to their inner world. Others (Bibring, 1959) note that the transient nature of pregnancy leads to avoidance by the therapist. Still others (Paluzny & Poznanski, 1971) note the tendency of the therapist to be less interested in the theoretical side of treatment.

No mention is made in the literature of the positive countertransference manifestations that may be evoked by the therapist's pregnancy. This might reflect a standard of the therapist as male. With that standard, the therapist's—or other women's issues—present only negative effects and problems. However, it would seem, and experience confirms, that the pregnant therapist might experience some positive effects in the treatment that is related to the pregnancy. The therapist's pregnancy can present an opportunity for the patient to mobilize ideation that leads to problem solving and resolution as well as to disruption and regression. Nadelson et al. (1974) points out that working through the conflicts around the therapist's pregnancy can be therapeutic for the patient. Similarly, although the therapist may find herself withdrawing energy from the therapeutic situation to her own body, she also may find that her empathic and intuitive resonance with patients is heightened as she becomes more sensitized to her own body. Although the scientific recedes, the irrational and emotional side of the process can become more available.

When the therapist consciously decides that the pregnancy *must* be dealt with in the treatment, several issues arise. These include when it should be brought up (if the patient persists in not noticing); how much should be discussed with the patient; and in what cases should the pregnancy be used as a corrective educational experience for the patient (i.e., discussing the mystique and miseducation about pregnancy). The answers to these questions depend upon the patient's developmental level. There are patients who will never bring up the therapist's pregnancy, as there are patients who do not bring up other topics without encouragement. There are patients for whom a passing comment might be sufficient and excessive dwelling might reflect the therapist's self-involvement rather than the interests and needs of the patient. Particularly important in the patient's history is the mother's pregnancy history with the patient and or siblings. Also developmentally important is whether or not the patient has children. Most important is the degree of the patient's pathology. Where the patient has difficulty distinguishing on any level between reality factors and transference factors, the most intense reaction to the pregnancy, and inversely the most intense denial, is likely to occur.

Whether the pregnancy remains a superficial topic in the treatment or a rallying point for many current and past fantasies, it is likely to evoke certain specific issues. Themes evoked include sibling rivalry, oedipal problems, separation anxiety, envy, sexuality, hostility and competition, and fear of abandonment.

Case Studies

An adaptation of categories developed by Paluzney & Poznanski (1971) are used to discuss the following cases. Patients' reactions to a therapist's pregnancy are divided into two groups: those for whom the pregnancy offers the opportunity for greater integration and those for whom the pregnancy results in greater disruption and regression. A distinction between the use of the material evoked by the therapist's pregnancy to deal with current life situations or to deal with problems rooted in early life circumstances also is made.

Case A. Integration and the Use of Material Evoked to Deal with Current Issues

A, a 28-year-old aspiring singer, came to treatment because of an incapacitating depression that was at times accompanied by suicidal thoughts. She had been unable to look for work for some time. At the start of treatment, she was a housewife for her husband and their cat. Her relationship with her husband was stormy, with loud angry fights, both verbal and physical. The fights seemed to have at their core competition and power issues. He was a successful businessman. When she became at all successful in singing (e.g., a performance with favorable reviews), he increased his demands for wifely services. When he was invited to a prestigious social event, she became too depressed to go.

A was the only child of immigrant parents. Her father had wished to be a singer but had become a successful lawyer instead. Her mother, a rather passive narcissistic woman, had made it her ambition to make *A* into a star. Dancing and singing lessons along with a great deal of grooming effort had made up her childhood. *A* was extremely pretty but felt that her prettiness was of no use. She stated: "People think that things come easily to you because you're pretty, but you never get anything really important from being pretty." It was not clear that *A* wanted to be a singer. She could not achieve much; she believed that only people like her husband or me, her therapist, could achieve. When she did achieve something, she immediately denigrated it. As the treatment progressed, she found herself more able to do things other than singing and the depression lifted somewhat. She and her husband both wanted a child and she attempted to conceive. After some time with no success, they found through medical tests that he had a problem which could be corrected by surgery.

During her fertility testing, she had a dream in which I appeared as her mother. With much prodding, she associated the dream to my pregnancy. She reacted with delight; she had noticed that I was getting heavier but had not wanted to mention it. During the course of my pregnancy, she spoke only of delight in it, how the pregnancy meant that she could have a baby also, etc. At the same time, the mother in her dreams turned into a dark, foreboding, witchlike character. Her associations revealed that she felt I was too powerful at times, both active and fecund, and therefore potentially destructive. That I did not become destructive and yet remained active was somewhat curative for her.

A's surface delight was congruent with her need to identify with me as the good, active mother. It was through this identification that she was able to give up her depression. (My pregnancy did not symbolize for her the birth of a sibling; sibling rivalry was not a significant issue in her life.) Shortly before treatment was terminated (prematurely because of her husband's job taking them to another city), she had a reinstatement of the depression and suicidal impulses that put her into a panic state. She telephoned me several times in great fear. Although I said very little to her on these calls, except to indicate that I was available to her, at the next session she reported that she felt she had really beat the depression. She had "let me in"; she would never be alone with the depression again. It was like living in a house alone; once you let somebody else in, you're never alone in it again. For this woman I was the benign identification model. When my pregnancy ended in a very late miscarriage, *A* reacted to the news with tears. By this time in the pregnancy, the "malevolent witch" was not appearing any longer for her. Although we explored her hostile wishes in relation to me and my pregnancy, what was most striking was the way in which she was able to use this experience to find her own strength. I had survived; she could survive and she could offer genuine sympathy.

Case B. Integration Through the Evoking of Primitive Associations.

B, a 26-year-old woman, has been treated for several years at a clinic. This previous treatment had been quite successful in helping her to go from an erratic work history to an advanced degree and a position of great responsibility in a large university. She had moved from her parents' home to an apartment of her own. Her relationships with people had changed. When she first began treatment she had hardly any significant relationships. Slowly she had developed a few rather distant but enduring ones. She had one woman friend and had begun a pursuit of men. Two "dates" with the same man were about all she could tolerate at the time she began her second treatment. Her aloneness and feeling of being shut out and peculiar were most apparent in her presentation of herself. This feeling had its roots in her parents' barely attending to her in favor of several other siblings, particularly a psychotic brother, several years her junior. Symbolic of this was her sleeping in her parents' living room because the psychotic brother refused to share a bedroom in the apartment with another brother. All of her siblings had a place in a bedroom; she alone slept in the living room.

B was one of the first patients to notice my pregnancy, which she came to through a dream about an older woman having a baby. Her immediate reaction was that I was foolish.

Why would a woman want to have a baby? She would get fat, become burdened, not be able to work or have fun, etc. This was presented in her characteristic bland, unrelated manner from which she went on to discuss the latest boyfriend and her problems having an orgasm.

Some time in the middle of the pregnancy, she noted that childbearing might not be too terrible if I were doing it. (I must have my reasons.) She informed me rather sadly that she did not think she could have children because of her problems. Towards the end of my pregnancy, when the presence of the "sibling" was very apparent and the ensuing separation had to be dealt with, *B* had a dream in which I was helping her decorate her apartment. With pain-racked sobs, she told me that if I had been her mother, I would have made a place for her (a room for her?) as I must be doing for my baby. I would not have allowed her to sleep in the living room. Her feelings about her apartment (rather sparsely furnished), her men, and her own body followed this discussion.

Most apparent in her relatedness to my pregnancy was her primitive identification with me as her mother, herself as baby, and the somewhat helpful use that she could make of it. Her relatedness to the pregnancy had much more transference than reality to it. It somehow provoked the deepest of pain for her and ultimately some resolution of it.

An interesting postscript was *B's* reaction to meeting me and my then 9-month-old daughter on the street (she lived in the same neighborhood). *B* stopped and made some nice comments on the child. During the next session, she spoke of how she felt it was important to me that she say nice things about the baby. She experienced her opinion to be valuable to me. Clearly, she was able to see herself related to me as another adult and not only her mother.

For both patients *A* and *B*, the pregnancy brought out some important problems and led to some resolution of them. For *B*, the reaction was much more intensely related to primitive associations to her mother. For *A*, who was much more related to the analyst as a real person, the reality elements of the pregnancy were more apparent and utilized by her.

Case C. Denial, Regression, and Flight

C, a 35-year-old man, was the oldest male child of four. He was much favored by his mother and ambivalently attached to her. His persistence in not noticing my pregnancy with yet another "sibling" reflected his difficulty with this ambivalence. When this pregnancy resulted in a late miscarriage, he almost immediately asked to use the couch. He insisted that it would be easier to talk while not facing me. He was able, therefore, to deny and isolate the fact of the pregnancy and the death of his hated sibling. Other important issues in his life—identification with his mother and pregnancy envy—could also thereby be avoided. These interpretations were not made to C. I erroneously believed that it was too soon in treatment for such interpretations. C left treatment soon after to take a business trip for several months. He came back in a panic from the interrupted trip because he had, in a rage that frightened him, almost killed a man who had cheated him in a business deal. Treatment resumed at that point with the connections made to the therapist and her baby as the hated objects that he wished to kill.

Case D. Disruption of Treatment to Handle the Intolerable

D, a 28-year-old graduate student in English literature, was in treatment with me during all of my four pregnancies. For her, birth was associated with death. She could not tolerate either pregnancies or miscarriages. The eldest of three sisters, she was supposed to "replace" an elder male sibling whom she had watched die as a young child. This replacement plus the death of a friend of hers during the first of my pregnancies, made my miscarriage intolerable for her. Her anger and hostility toward me, as well as her guilt for the death of the fetus, was too much for her to face. She left treatment for 6 months, by which time she assumed it would all be over. The second pregnancy, (resulting in an early miscarriage) went unnoticed by her. During the next pregnancy, she took a trip out of town, to return when it was over and baby and mother were home safely. During the fourth of my pregnancies, she stayed until I took leave, but called me several days after my leave began in great depression. Her mother had become ill, which was too much for her to deal with at that time. This telephone contact with her during my leave seemed to reassure her that I was still alive and available. She resumed treatment after the birth of my second child, somewhat better able to look at her depressions and regression, but never quite able to get to her deeper feelings about pregnancy, childbirth, and death.

For both patients, C and D, my pregnancies were intolerable, and resulted in enormous disruption and regression. Certainly there might have been better ways to deal with these patients so that flight did not occur. The important point is, however, that the pregnancy of the therapist was the occurrence that led to the greater disruption and potential disorganization of the patient.

The cases presented are meant to be illustrative, not prototypic. From them, we can see that as each patient presents a unique history and constellation of reactions, so it is the case with their relationship to the therapist's pregnancy. Reactions vary as much as reactions to the therapist herself vary. Similarly, countertransference issues will differ for each therapist. The "real" personality of the therapist as always, will have its effect. For one therapist it is the stormy angry feelings of the patient that are the most difficult to relate to, for another, the tender protective feelings evoked in the patient may be intolerable.

In general, the pregnancy of the therapist evokes complicated reactions in treatment and strains the therapist's understanding and skill. Several things are important. The pregnancy must be noted, explored at different stages of the pregnancy, and allowed to flourish as an issue for discussion and an outgrowth of the patient's history. Some decision about how long she will work has to be made by the therapist and communicated to the patients, whether or not they ask. Some decision about how much reality will be shared with patients must be made by the therapist, e.g. the date of birth, sex of child, nature of labor, etc. How much the therapist uses her pregnancy as an "educational" experience for patients, where applicable, has to be decided. These questions need to be answered individually by each therapist faced with them. The answers may vary according to the history of the patient and should have as their goal the facilitation of treatment.

Concerning miscarriage, Cain et al. (1974) show the neglect of the topic in standard textbooks of obstetrics and psychiatry. Considering the high incidence of miscarriage, this is striking. There is only one article (Hannett, 1949) that deals with an analyst's miscarriage. The analyst did not tell her patients that the reason for her absence was her miscarriage. She left it for them to surmise or not. Cain et al. discussed children's reactions to their mother's miscarriages, which are similar to patients' reactions to a therapist's miscarriage. An initial puzzlement, followed by guilt over the hostile thought towards the fetus that magically came true, guilt over envy of the therapist, and blame of the therapist for having actively "killed" her baby. Surely if the therapist could not carry a fetus to birth, she could not be an adequate mother to the patient. Along with these reactions are also the fears of childbearing that women patients have that get exaggerated. For male patients, all of the discomfort, fear, awe, and disgust that they feel toward women's insides get stirred up. For some, there is little deep meaning, for others very deep transferential issues come up leading to a period of chaos and hopefully resolution. The reactions vary, as do the reactions to the pregnancy itself, from minimal transient ones to enduring profound effects.

The long-term effect of the therapist's pregnancy on the treatment of a particular individual would be difficult to measure. My observations indicate that it can and should be used as a productive event in the treatment. Although it should be clear that great turmoil and disruption can occur, skill and creative handling of the situation can lead to movement in the treatment that might have otherwise not occurred.

REFERENCES

Balsam, R., & Balsam, A. *Becoming a therapist.* Boston: Little Brown, 1974.

Benedek, E. P. The fourth world of the pregnant therapist. *Journal American Medical Womens Association,* 1973, *28,* 365–368.

Bibring, G. L. Some considerations of the psychological processes in pregnancy. *Psychoanalytic Study of the Child,* 1959, *14,* 113–122.

Bibring, G. L., Dwyer, T. F., Huntington, D. S. & Valenstein, A. F. A study of the psychological processes in pregnancy and of the earliest mother-child relationship. *Psychoanalytic Study of the Child,* 1961, *16,* 9–73.

Browning, D. H. Patients' reactions to their therapist's pregnancies. *Journal American Academy of Child Psychiatry,* 1974, *13,* 468–482.

Cain, A. C., Erickson, M. E., Fast, I., & Vaughan, R. A. Children's disturbed reactions to their mother's miscarriage. *Psychosomatic Medicine,* 1964, *26* N (1), 58–67.

Hannett, F. Transference reactions to an event in the life of the analyst. *Psychoanalytic Review,* 1949, *36,* 69–81.

Klein, H. Pregnancy and childbirth. In Masserman, J. (Ed.). *Progress in psychotherapy,* vol. *2,* New York, Grune & Stratton, 1957, 98–103.

Klein, H., Potter, H., & Dyk, R. *Anxiety in pregnancy and childbirth.* New York: Paul B. Haeber, 1950.

Lax, R. F. Some considerations about transference and countertransference manifestations evoked by the analyst's pregnancy. *International Journal of Psychoanalysis,* 1969, *50,* 363–372.

Le Bow, M. Paper presented at the 1963 Psychoanalytic Mid-Winter Meeting, New York City.

Nadelson, C., Notman, J., Arons, E., & Feldman, J. The pregnant therapist. *American Journal of Psychiatry,* 1974, *131* (10), 1107–1111.

Paluzny, M., & Poznanski, E. Reactions of patients during pregnancy of the psychotherapist. *Child Psychiatry and Human Development,* 1971, *1* (4), 266–274.

Schwartz, M. D. Casework implications of a worker's pregnancy. *Social Casework,* 1975, *56,* 27–34.

Stone, L. *The psychoanalytic situation.* New York: International Universities Press, 1961.

Part III

BIRTHING AND BONDING

Some describe giving birth as a peak experience, an "oceanic high," while others regard it as a transitional stage in an ongoing relationship with a child. In either case, experiences during and immediately following labor and delivery can have long-lasting ramifications for the infant, mother, and the family as a whole. The contributors to this section consider the family's psychological as well as functional/medical needs during this period. The rationale for current birthing procedures in hospitals and their potential effects on the psychological, physical, and cognitive well-being of the child and parents is explored. Alternatives are proposed. Also discussed are the special psychological needs of families coping with stillbirths or ill neonates.

chapter 15

A PSYCHOHISTORICAL VIEW OF 19TH AND 20TH CENTURY BIRTH PRACTICES

Alice Eichholz

Control of birth services has changed hands several times throughout history. Originally the province of the mother and midwife, it later became the responsibility of the developing medical profession in the United States. Finally, it entered the sphere of the hospital, where drugs and technology predominately controlled the process, guided by the 20th century obstetrician.

Recently, birth services in the United States have had a dual direction. The first is toward home birth and family-centered maternity care, which many have seen as a frightening, emotional regression into the past, while others see it as a way for women to regain control of their own natural bodily processes. The second direction is toward complete obstetric management including drugs, machines, and surgery. None of these developments are accidents of history. Central to each has been the individual woman—her psyche, fears, joys—her unconscious. The woman's psychology has had a profound effect on the course of birth services.

It is difficult in historical research to speculate about the unconscious of the past. But there are clues both from the present and past. Three major points of transition all extending over long periods of time are apparent in the history of birth practices. The change from female midwife to male midwife and later physician; the relocation of the birth scene from home to the lying-in hospital and then from lying-in hospital to technological management within neonatal centers in medical facilities. At present, another period of transition appears possible— from technological management to family-centered birth without violence. This last period, only begun recently, is far from over. Looking at these developments from a slightly different perspective may help to understand what happened underneath the changes in the past. At present

> Doctors retain control of birth and most patients are rendered powerless in the experience. While women welcome [more humanizing birth] most still defer to medical judgment about medicalization and would find any other arrangement unthinkable. Women are largely eager and passive consumers of medicine, depending upon doctors, drugs and hospitals to produce health for themselves and their children rather than depending on themselves and on inner strength of natural process. Most women therefore acquiese in the view of birth as potential disease. (Wertz & Wertz, 1977, pp. 235–236)

The history of childbirth services contains an interesting contradiction. As women have historically become more emancipated, the choices they make in birth experiences appear to be more and more removed from a natural, normal, internal process to one where the control is not only put predominately in the hands of a person of another sex, but in the control of asexual mechanical devices which give the illusion of protection and safety, but, in reality, may be quite the opposite.

During the three major changes, the birth experience also moved further and further away from one where the woman had little anatomic knowledge of herself, to one where the knowledge was available, but where it was invested in others, outside of, rather than inside, herself. Woman have deferred to the outsider's control because of a probable, persistent underlying unconscious feeling that to do otherwise was to risk death, not necessarily in the literal sense, but in the sense of finally breaking the symbiosis with their own mothers.

The fact that men (gynecologists and the entire medical team) have capitalized on women's fear, and added to it their own desires for power, authority, and money is not entirely their own fault. "Because there are so many more frightened than composed pregnant women (and frightened women who appear composed), the attendant, by reason of the transference that obtains during gestation and labor, has enormous influence to assuage or to intensify anxiety" (Rheingold, 1966, p. 537). Power relationships are always two-way affairs as Albert Memmi has clearly described in his books *Dominated Man* (1968) and *The Colonizer and the Colonized* (1975). Women, at every stage of the transition, have bought the righteousness of that authority for their own psychological reasons. One such reason is the possibility of unconsciously choosing to remain dependent, passive, and compliant because it keeps them from having to surpass their mothers and break the symbiotic tie.

This suggestion, often found in psychoanalytic literature, also is reflected in the history of birth services. During the 19th century, there were a variety of services available: midwives both male and female; a variety of medical practitioners; and various birthing places such as home, borning rooms, and lying-in hospitals. The rules and regulations of 20th century medicine and technological control were not yet operative. Yet, increasingly, women, as a group, turned away from their own sense of control. There were, of course, exceptions. Elizabeth Cady Stanton tried to encourage women to look to their own inner strengths. In 1891, in Saur's *Maternity,* she stated, as cited by Wertz and Wertz, (1977):

What an incubus it would take from woman could she be educated to know that the pains of maternity are no curse upon her
kind . . . But one word of fact is worth a volume of philosphy;
let me give you some of my own experience. I am the mother of
seven children. My girlhood was spent mostly in the open air.
I early imbibed the idea that *a girl is just as good as a boy,* and
I carried it out. I would walk five miles before breakfast . . . wore
my clothing sensibly . . . never compressed my body . . . When
my first four children were born, I suffered very little. I then
made up my mind that it was totally unnecessary for me to suffer
at all; so I dressed lightly, walked every day . . . The night before
the birth . . . I walked three miles. The child was born *without
a particle of pain.* I bathed it and dressed it myself. (p. 115).

Wertz and Wertz (1977) suggest that the rationale behind
each woman's personal choice for childbirth procedures was
social class. Social class, however, does not seem to be enough
of an explanation. There is a possibility that some of that choosing had to do with how women viewed themselves individually.
Those views derived from their own childhood and their relationship with their mothers.

Present day services, to some extent, offer a choice to
women. Yet, in large numbers, women continue to choose the
neonatal facilities with the vast extent of technological support.
While it is true that profit has been an important motive of
the medical profession, to maintain technological control, no
conscious or unconscious motive seems so obvious in the history of birth practices as that of anxiety and fear. Anxiety, a
heightened sense of unknown danger, produces fears of loss,
injury, and death. In the 17th and 18th century, there was much
less physiological knowledge about the birth process, but most
people, especially women, had more actual experience. Women
were closer to the realities of birth because of the circumstances
of colonial and rural life. Now women take childbirth classes,
tour hospitals, and watch movies and read books in order to
gain some personal experience for their first pregnancy. One
could almost suggest that the recent abundance of popular
literature is an attempt, through the written word, for women

to create the social birth of shared experience with other women, which many say existed in the past.

Pain is a concomitant reality to anxiety and fear. It is not easy to know whether women in the 17th and 18th century experienced birth pain to the same extent that 19th and 20th century women apparently do. It seems quite probable that the "advancements" of a technological society have increased pain. The original birth position of standing; walking until the final stage; squatting on a birth stool for transition, birth, and after birth makes enormous sense physiologically for two reasons: gravity is put to work and pain is always less with freedom of movement.

The two most popular "advancements" certainly would have increased the pain of childbirth both physically and psychologically. When Louis XIV had his wife's physician devise an examining table from which they could both view the birth process without either making eye contact with the expectant mother, the procedure became the rage of the upper classes and over the next 200 years became universally used. Women were put flat on their backs, a position which common sense would note was not the best, but a position which reinforced submissiveness, passivity, dependency, and a sense of illness with accompanying pain.

The second most popular development in obstetric management were the straps. They came in various shapes, sizes, and with varying purposes but they all were ways of tying down and containing. These included uterine supports, pessaries in the mid-1800s to keep the uterus from falling out, and corsets in the Victorian era to hold the abdomen in and to keep the outside world from knowing that the woman participated in sexual intercourse and was not "pure." Stirrups and straps in the 1920s to keep a woman from interfering with the process, fetal heart monitors with, at first, belts surrounding the contracting abdomen and later an electrode screwed into the infant's skull in utero and connected by a cord to a machine have been used. These later devices, which are standard operating procedures in many hospitals, appear to have increased the percentage of cesarean sections performed.

Symbolically, these devices appear to have one purpose outside of the medical rationale: something is collapsing, weak, dying, and must be saved. Walls, borders, and boundaries need to be stabilized. It is time for structure to make sure that things do not collapse. Women have given over the control of that structuring and become great consumers of medical structure possibly because of the unconscious fear of their own mothers, symbolically dying, with the birth of their own child. The birthing woman is taking her mother's place. To resolve the conflict felt about such an occurence, splitting between the good mother and the bad mother ought take place. The pregnant woman might incorporate the "damaged, sick, ill" bad mother, maintaining the symbiosis with her own mother. To do this is adaptive. The doctor, then, becomes the good mother with the right tools, equipment and, for the most part, sex to make the transference safe. "The good mother image [molding oneself after a nurturant mother] and the acceptance of pregnancy too often succumb to the need of safety created by [threats from] the bad mother image which calls forth, potential death, mutilation, or destructive fantasies" (Rheingold, 1964, p. 534). It is important to understand that endowing the doctor or birth attendant with a good mother image makes the woman a good patient in the doctor's eyes.

Some definition of self which maintains the symbiotic fantasy and, that especially when threatened maintains the borders on boundaries, is critically important. Those boundaries, in the instance of pregnancy, can be viewed as the increasing size and contractions of the uterus. Especially during the second stage of labor, the fear of the body's boundaries bursting is quite common. There may be an inner pressure at work to maintain the borders, not let things get out of hand, make the situation more controlled and "like" others and therefore be "normal." The shared fantasy projected by the medical community may be that they are the protectors of the borders between life and death, and also protectors of the symbiotic borders. They play a role in maintaining the symbiosis at a point of crisis. The woman struggling to maintain herself even in the most physical terms is a threat to that symbiosis.

In fact, during the 1920s, another "advancement" in technology allowed this projection and protection to continue to a greater extent. The medical community began to promise to prevent pain and tragedy. Twilight sleep and other anesthetics which rendered women unaware of the entire birth process were not only advertized, but some hospitals and many women adopted them eagerly. As with the use of the constraining equipment and procedures which may have increased pain rather than diminished it, the use of hospitalization and drugs has not prevented tragedy. In too many cases, the price paid is the tragedy that was supposed to have been averted. For example, when birthing was moved into the hospital, many deaths and injuries resulted from puerperal fever. Also, drugs and anesthesia have been shown to cause birth injury. But, if women were put to sleep during birth, control and the "normalcy" of the process was maintained. One delivery could be very similiar to the next, even to the amount of time it would take. In fact, one argument used today for the use of the fetal heart monitor is just that. Since the birth process is so unexpected and unpredictable, the monitor acts as a control to make each birth more alike and therefore more manageable. What that management has resulted in as mentioned previously, has been more cesarean section deliveries. With the exception of a small number of doctors and expectant parents who have begun to challenge these basic assumptions prevalent in birth services, it would appear that the final extention of control, similarity of delivery, and maintanence of the symbiotic relationship with passive-dependent patients is the use of test tube babies and the fantasy of cloning, so close on the horizon of birth services.

If the course of birth services is to take a different direction, one that is toward humanistic birth, two things would have to happen. First, women will have to decide that they want humanistic childbirth. Without the consumer, the medical profession would not have the opportunity to sell their technology. Second, the medical profession will have to be open to new ways of trying to come to terms with the uniqueness of each birth experience. Further, childbirth must be viewed as neither a disease or illness.

Many interesting approaches to more individualized humanistic birth that attempt to work with the medical profession have begun to emerge. Organizations supporting home births, birthing centers, and humanistic hospital based birth experiences have formed and are providing experiential and research data to prospective parents.[1] Psychologists, social workers, nurses, and childbirth educators have joined with physicians and midwives to help expectant parents look at alternative birth practices and to guide individuals and couples to a clearer understanding of their own needs, expectations, and fantasies about the birth of their children. Perhaps a greater understanding of the determinants of childbirth methods will contribute to more individualized and more humanistic childbirth experiences.

REFERENCES

Memmi, A. *Dominated man.* Boston: Beacon Press, 1968.
Memmi, A. *The colonizer and the colonized.* New York: Viking Press, 1975.
Rheingold, J. *Fear of being a woman: A theory of maternal destructiveness* New York: Grune & Stratton, 1964.
Rheingold, J. *Mother anxiety and death.* Boston: Little Brown, 1967.
Wertz, R., & Wertz, R. *Lying in: A history of childbirth in America.* New York: Free Press, 1977.

[1]For information about this direction see material from the National Association of Parents and Professionals for Safe Alternatives in Childbirth (NAPSAC). Chapel Hill, North Carolina or the International Childbirth Education Association, P.O. Box 20852 Milwaukee, Wisc. 53220. See also LeBoyer, F. *Birth without violence.* New York: Knopf, 1975.

chapter 16

DESIGNING AN ENVIRONMENT FOR CHILDBIRTH
An Architect's Approach

William A. Parker, Jr.

Many women are approaching delivery with a better understanding of their physiological and psychological needs during childbirth. Husbands are present during labor and delivery, and families are increasingly concerned about the use of drugs or anesthesia. People are beginning to question whether the hospital is the most appropriate setting, or if the harsh lights and sterilized bustle should be replaced with a more home-like environment.

Khalifa Mishri

There is considerable public dissatisfaction with the current health care delivery system—the lack of personal attention, increasing costs, the unevenness in quality, accessibility and availability of care. These problems are not limited to the United States; they are worldwide, even though organizational models vary from country to country depending on culture and tradition. The systems for providing obstetrical care must take into consideration the economic and sociological factors of the communities being served, and must be coordinated with other components in the health care delivery system. The importance of historical patterns in seeking out medical assistance is often greater than we imagine.

Yolanda Alvarez

The literature suggests that two approaches exist for childbirth. One is born out of the medical disease model of health and argues for a high degree of surgical intervention. The other more traditional view argues for a totally natural process with little or no medical intervention. Today's concern for individual rights and the rights of patients makes the natural process appealing, but unfortunately both approaches argue as if the two extremes are the only possible choices. It is not inconceivable that a range of environmental experiences needs to be provided in order for mothers to have access to the care they need. I would expect different mothers, often with the advice of a physician or midwife, to feel that they need different types of care experiences during pregnancy and at birth. Either the medical interventionist or natural childbirth approach may force conditions onto mothers and families that may not always be desirable.

Philip Allsopp

This chapter takes a fresh look, from the architect's perspective, at the design of the obstetrics and delivery environment in the hospital setting. A conceptual methodology for evaluating the spatial and environmental needs of an obstetrics and delivery department is proposed. Areas for additional design investigation are suggested, and specific design approaches are recommended.

The work presented here is based on design studio investigations done in January and February of 1979 in the Health Services Planning and Design Program in the Graduate School of Architecture and Planning at Columbia University. Significant contributions are included from the following three graduate students: Philip Allsopp, R.I.B.A., from England; Yolanda Alvarez, from Venezuela; Khalifa Mishri, from Libya.

BACKGROUND

Throughout most of this century, reproduction of the species has existed within the hospital. The medical specialities have made great advances in their understanding of the human body and the diseases that affect it, and the amount and complexity of information about childbrith has grown tremendously. New facilities and techniques have been developed to ease delivery and provide better information on the condition of the child. As general anesthesia became a widely available method of reducing pain, it quickly won the popular support of both obstetricians and expectant mothers. Through the use of new monitoring equipment, we are now learning more about the physical well-being of the baby during childbirth. The design of obstetrics and delivery facilities has tried to accommodate the latest medical and technical expertise to ensure the safest possible level of care for both mother and child. "Safety" and "reduction of pain" have been the predominant criteria of this medical approach to childbirth.

As we learn more about childbirth, the design criteria for the labor and delivery environments are being forced to reflect a major reorientation: childbirth is now becoming regarded once again as a natural process, not as a disease. Society is providing better prenatal care, better screening techniques, and better education for expectant mothers. As a result, the need for highly technical and specialized facilities, previously designed specifically for the delivery department, has been reduced. Natural childbirth techniques open a world of information to the expecting mother, teaching her about her body and the process she will experience, providing natural methods for dealing with pain instead of relying on anesthesia or drugs. As a result, environments for childbirth need to be less procedure-oriented and more sensitive to social and psychological needs.

The two paragraphs above reveal two dramatically different points of view concerning childbirth. One sees childbirth as a "pathologic" process; the other sees it as a "natural" process. Taken as extremes, the two points of view result in the following functional, social, and environmental characteristics:

PATHOLOGIC	*NATURAL*
Medical/surgical intervention	Psychosocial assistance
General anesthesia	Psychoprophylaxis
Dependence	Independence
Restraint	Mobility
Surgical environment	Homelike environment
Medical equipment	Residential furniture
Hard, "clean" finishes	Soft finishes
Tile floor	Carpet

The apparent incompatibility of these characteristics illustrates the difficulties encountered when designing an environment for labor and delivery. How can an environment be designed to meet the functional needs of the staff but not jeopardize the psychological needs of the mother, father, and newborn? The real concerns about cross-contamination, isolation, and cleanliness must be met, but they cannot be allowed to result in an environment having the aesthetic appeal of a public bathroom.

The architectural design process is one of giving physical form to the functional and environmental objectives and goals of the space users. The symbolic and perceptual richness of any design can be traced back to the functions being accommodated and the social and psychological context surrounding those functions. If a balance between functional and social design criteria is not achieved, then the resulting environment will be distorted or idiosyncratic. A predominance of functional criteria in the design process may result in a "factory" or a "machine" for childbirth. A predominance of social or perceptual design criteria could result in a "home" or a "lounge." Both examples represent exaggerated environments, and each could result in a biased and inflexible department.

The context surrounding the obstetrics and delivery department is going through some dramatic changes. Public attitudes about health care in general are evolving, and current aggressive attempts to modify the obstetrics and delivery environment can be seen as part of a broader desire to make the environment of today's hospitals less institutional and more sensitive to the perceptual and psychological needs of the patient. Before attempting to "deinstitutionalize" the hospital environment, some investigative design research should be done to determine which qualities of those environments make them "institutional." A building design may be considered institutional when functional criteria preclude satisfaction of social need, or when the typical requirements of user groups (patients, staff, etc.) unnecessarily limit the number of options available to individuals. However, in order to provide a responsive, sensitive, and meaningful environment for the potentially wide range of activities and needs experienced by today's expecting mother, the department design must not preclude a correspondingly wide range of perceptual and behavioral options. Every mother is different and will experience childbirth differently. Each mother will therefore have different physical and psychosocial needs, and should be able to find the appropriate amount and kind of support (medical or social) from her labor/delivery environment. The first child for an unwed 18-year-old could be frightening, while the third child for a mother trained in natural childbirth could be routine. While a natural childbirth enthusiast should not be forced into a rigid pathologic process, a frightened young mother may be reassured by the technical expertise it offers. The design of a labor and delivery facility should be able to accommodate both mothers and the wide variation in behavior that may be expected. The design should not preclude a mother opting for either of the two extremes, or for some comfortable yet reassuring combination of social and medical support.

FUNCTIONAL PROFILE

Admitting

Perhaps the most critical function to consider in the design of an obstetrics and delivery department is the initial admitting process. When entering the hospital, a person goes through the transition from being Ms. Somebody to being patient XYZ. The admittee surrenders her personal belongings to the hospital, and puts on the institution's gown and I.D. bracelet (just in case they forget her name). Symbolically, she gives up some of her individuality when she turns over control of her care to the hospital (Taylor, 1970). If the admission space is an anonymous room, or a chair in the hall, then her insignificance is reinforced. The ticket window or admitting booth design can also make the admittee feel somewhat transient. As an alternative, a small admitting office provides privacy and lends a formal sense of importance to the admitting interview, thereby reinforcing the patient's individual identity.

When a woman is admitted to an obstetrics and delivery department, she is "prepped." This procedure normally consists of a shower, a pubic shave, and the starting of I.V. fluids. The mysteries of what goes on behind the closed doors of the prep room have been cited by several observers (Rosengren & DeVault, 1963) as intimidating or even frightening. The "prep" processes can be routinized to the extent that it is a dehumanizing experience and greatly reinforces the individual identity-robbing quality of checking into the hospital. It can be a much less negative experience if prepping activities are conducted in the mother's bedroom.

A mother should have her own home base while she's in the hospital. Her bedroom should be her own individual territory upon which she may place her own stamp of identity, making it her own. This should be established as early as possible. By transferring both the admitting and prepping activities into her room, a mother is symbolically put in a position of control rather than total dependence. Her individuality is reinforced, and the first step is taken to reduce the institutional quality of the childbirth experience.

Labor

The first stage of labor can be quite prolonged (8 to 10 hours) and experienced with widely varying degrees of discomfort. Many women will go through a large portion of the first stage of labor at home where they can relax in familiar surroundings, walk around, and talk with friends. It's quite common, however, for mothers to arrive at the hospital prematurely, resulting in a prolonged 15-hour stay in the labor room. During this time, she may want to be alone with her husband, or she may prefer to walk and socialize with family or friends. In fact, some physicians encourage mothers to stay mobile as long as possible. Options should therefore be available to the mother. If privacy is wanted, she remains in her room (home base). If she opts for social support and mobility, then there should be a lounge or gallery for her to stroll or sit in with friends.

Some of the equipment and techniques used to monitor the fetus during labor can restrict a patient's mobility. Normally, the physician or nurse will monitor the strength and spacing of the mother's contractions as well as of the baby's heartbeat. If a baby goes into distress, they want to know about it as soon as possible in order to take the necessary life-saving steps. Monitor leads are normally attached to the mother by a padded belt that she wears across her abdomen, and the monitoring equipment sits beside the bed. As long as she's "plugged in," she is generally restricted to her bed. Technical equipment requirements can often dominate the use or quality of hospital environments, and it is very important for a mother to understand the advantages and limitations of the equipment, and to know what options exist. Can she take off the belt and stand up for a moment? If it would be more comfortable, can she sit in a chair? Many of these issues will be discussed with her physician or the nursing staff, but the design of the bedroom should allow for these options without limiting the effectiveness of the monitoring equipment. Hopefully, improved equipment and the use of telemetry will allow both continuous monitoring and mobility during labor.

During the second stage of labor, and particularly during the final hour before delivery, most women experience pain. The typical reaction to pain is a need for privacy and/or medical support. The mother's room should continue to serve as home base during this potentially dramatic portion of the childbirth process. The father may become very important during this time, particularly if he has been trained in natural childbirth techniques. On the other hand, the mother may simply want to be alone. It is very likely, however, that the mother's and father's focus will shift from the social support of a lounge to the medical support of the staff work area or nurse station. A very significant transition could occur: the shift from a feeling of competence to a feeling of dependence on the support of the medical staff.

Delivery

Most normal deliveries do not require the antiseptic environment of the typical delivery room and could therefore occur in the mother's bedroom, provided there is adequate space for staff and equipment. For many deliveries, the delivery table position (on the back with the feet in the air) is neither comfortable nor physiologically helpful to the mother. The process of pushing the baby out can be naturally assisted by gravity if the mother is in a sitting or reclining position. The hospital bed can be much more comfortable, and some new designs allow the foot of the bed to be lowered for better access to the baby during delivery. Some mothers find the traditional delivery room environment, with all of its technical equipment-dominated aesthetic, symbolically and psychologically reassuring. However, many women find it mechanical, frightening, and more like a torture chamber than a warm environment in which to deliver a baby.

Unfortunately, medical knowledge and skills have not been able to eliminate all of the risks associated with childbirth. Although much less frequent than 30 years ago, maternal deaths still do occur. Compared to other highly developed countries, the United States still has a relatively high perinatal death rate. Childbirth is a very unpredictable process, and there will always be a need for emergency medical support services for both mother and child. Occasionally, surgical intervention is necessary during delivery. The mother must be moved as quickly as possible to a surgical room, which should be immediately available to all delivery locations. Also, intensive care or premature nurseries with isolation capabilities must be immediately available for babies in distress. New information and ideas concerning childbirth will continue to evolve, and although there is a clear demand for the design of delivery facilities which are less technologically dominant, less complex, less frightening, and more comfortable or homelike, emergency medical backup services must be provided.

Recovery

After delivery of the baby and a brief exam, the mother and father may want a quiet moment together with their child. Perhaps an hour or two to be alone, to get acquainted, to count the baby's toes and fingers, and to relax might be necessary. They are now a family and may need some time to adjust. The delivery environment should be conducive to the quiet nature of this recovery period; and, in fact, that time could be spent in the mother's bedroom or home base.

The majority of normal deliveries can occur entirely in the mother's bedroom. Labor, delivery, and recovery can all happen in the same room if that room is designed and equipped to accommodate all the needs of the mother, the baby, the father, the physician, the nurse, and support staff. A mother does not have to be moved from room to room as she progresses from the first stage of labor to the second stage, from labor to delivery, and so on. In fact, that routine or circuit can be disorienting to the mother and leave her feeling like a cog in a machine. It certainly does not contribute to a sense of individuality, or allow a mother to develop a "home base" and the accompanying sense of personal territory.

After the quiet recovery period, a mother may be moved

into a more typical patient bedroom, often a multiple bedroom, for a short stay in the hospital. If, however, she could remain in a private room for the 2 or 3 days that she and the baby may stay in the hospital, then it would be possible for the father to stay the night with them. Childbirth is, after all, a natural process with major significance to the family unit, and the design of environments for childbirth should be able to accommodate fathers, siblings, and other relatives. The active participation of other family members, particularly the father, during childbirth can provide important social and psychological support to the mother, and the design and configuration of obstetrics and delivery departments must not limit their access or participation.[1]

Design Concepts

The functional profile above describes a concept commonly known as the "birthing room," a single room designed to accommodate labor, delivery, and recovery. Birthing rooms have been added to many existing obstetrics/delivery departments by enlarging several labor rooms and changing the furnishings. The quality of the resulting environment is described in the following quote.

> Late-afternoon sunshine streams through the flower-patterned curtains, casting a warm, soft light on the hanging plants and queen-size brass bed. There's classical music in the air and a dinner on a side table. Leaning against a beanbag chair on the bed, Diane Boutcher nurses her newborn son, Joseph, as her husband James sits beside her, gently stroking the baby's black hair. The family will sleep together here tonight. The cozy room where Joseph Boutcher was born is at Illinois Masonic Medical

[1]Thanks to Dr. John Dwyer, Department of Obstetrics and Gynecology of Roosevelt Hospital, New York City, and to Ms. Elisabeth Bing, childbirth educator and co-founder of the American Society of Psychoprophylaxis in Obstetrics, Inc., New York, for discussing these concepts.

Center. It is part of the hospitals' Alternative Birthing Center, a radically different setting for labor and delivery. Neither medical equipment nor drugs are used routinely here. A mother may give birth assisted by her spouse, other relatives or friends, a nurse-midwife—or even the baby's brothers and sisters. Use of the center costs about half as much as a conventional delivery, and couples can enjoy a relaxed, homelike birth within the safe confines of a fully equipped hospital. If complications arise, a woman is quickly moved down the hall to the regular delivery room.

(Lublin, 1979 p.1)

That description suggests an environment which is much less institutional than the majority of existing obstetrics and delivery departments, and it also suggests that the birthing room is becoming more widely accepted as an alternative to those traditional environments. One ususally finds the birthing room with the "regular" delivery facilities down the hall. But, what happens if the birthing room is considered the "regular" delivery location, with the emergency facilities just down the hall? How can the childbirth environment be designed to accommodate the wider range of demands being placed on it? How can one provide all of the necessary emergency and medical support, but not let them dominate the perceptual quality of the environment? If 90 to 95 percent of all births occur within the birthing room, how should that room be designed and what other facilities are necessary?

The birthing room is the conceptual center of the labor/-delivery environment and home base for the mother—her individual territory. Diagramatically, the mother should be at the center of a range or field of support services. On one side she has access to the social and psychological support of family and friends. She can go out to them or invite them into the birthing room. On the other side, she has access to medical and nursing support; and again, she can reach out to them or call them to her bedside. She also has immediate access to emergency and-/or surgical support services should they be necessary (Fig. 16-1).

When the figure is expanded to investigate the spatial organization or structure of activities, distinct zones appear. The social and family support zone is the least specific, with lounges, waiting areas, conversation alcoves, and gallery spaces for short walks. At the center is the birthing room environment, accessi-

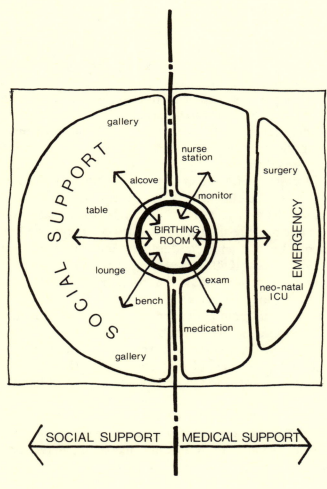

Fig. 16-1.

ble from the social areas on one side and from the medical support zone on the other side. The segregation of activities is defined in terms of the continuum above the figure. Moving from left to right, one moves from the most public and social spaces to the most private medical spaces with restricted entry. The quality of the spaces is very general on the left, becoming more specific as one moves to the right, and the relative roles of the mother, father, and medical staff change as one moves through these zones. On the left, one can imagine the mother as being in control, completely competent in childbirth. On the right, the mother becomes totally dependent upon the medical expertise of the emergency staff and facilities.

Figure 16-2 also suggests the options available to a mother and father as they enter the department for the birth of their child. They may check in with some of the staff and spend several hours in the lounge or gallery area. As the mother's contractions get stronger, she may want to move into the birthing room, and if everything goes normally she will deliver her baby in that room with the assistance of the medical and nursing support staff. If complications develop, a mother may move into a traditional delivery room or even into a surgical environment for a cesarean section delivery. The full range of support services is structured into four zones, and a mother penetrates the zones as needed. A mother experiencing an easy labor and a normal childbirth would only move into the central zone— the birthing room (home base). If emergency procedures are required, then the mother would penetrate further into zone 4 where she becomes totally dependent upon the medical staff.

The objective is to spatially organize the full range of social and medical support activities in a manner which maximizes a mother's access to the level of support she needs, yet does not preclude any reasonable option. The frightened mother should be able to lean on the medical support in zones 3 or 4 as much as she needs, but the natural childbirth enthusiast should be able to remain in the lounge to the last minute. The mother going through a prolonged labor in the birthing room can change her focus from the social support on the zone 1 side to

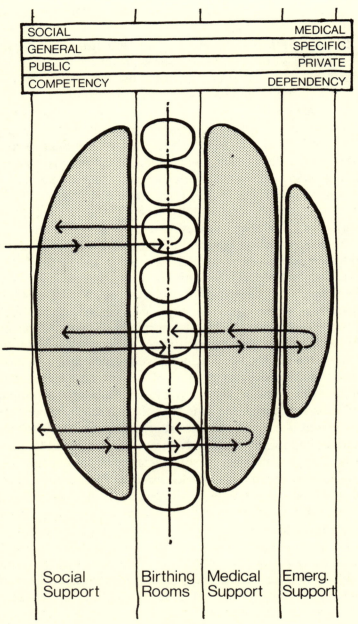

SOCIAL — MEDICAL
GENERAL — SPECIFIC
PUBLIC — PRIVATE
COMPETENCY — DEPENDENCY

Social Support   Birthing Rooms   Medical Support   Emerg. Support

Fig. 16-2.

270

the medical support on the zone 3 side, and back again if that's what she needs. The birthing room, zone 2, is still the central element in the entire range of environments and serves as the mother's home base. She's at the center, in control (although maybe with considerable medical support) with access to everything she needs.

The division of the diagram into zones also implies that there are distinct separations between activities. Segregation of functions, or the prohibition of certain activities in specific spaces, is quite common in hospitals. "You can't do that in here!" "Children are not allowed in this room!" "This patient should be transferred to another room." This type of segregation of activities is usually a direct result of functional and/or medical considerations, and it can both isolate incompatible activities (both medically and socially) and indiscriminately segregate naturally related activities.

The traditional use of space to routinize the labor and delivery process is quite clear. The labor room—delivery room —recovery room—laying-in room sequence tends to formalize, through the use of space, the childbirth process. The strict segregation of medical activities or phases of childbirth into separate rooms limits the flexibility and therefore the options available to the mother, particularly if she is interested in a more natural childbirth.

The birthing room is a specific attempt to combine, in a single room, compatible activities which have traditionally been segregated into three or four spaces. Because of its location, as described in Figure 16-2, the birthing room zone can also be characterized as an edge between the social activities on one side and the medical activities on the other side. The birthing room is the important dividing element that separates or modulates those activities, but it is also a very important "place." It is the place where a majority of mothers will deliver their babies. The birthing room is an edge or transitional space and, at the same time, the single most important place in the entire department. It's an *interstitial space,* but its functions are the central purpose of the entire department.

The notion of interstitial space with special functional significance is an important departure from current architectural vocabularies. A corridor is an example of an interstitial space. It provides access to other functional spaces, but it generally has no formal significance in the building's purpose. It is the services space which is necessary for the functional space to be useful (Sommer, 1969).[2] The behavior patterns in interstitial spaces tend to be less rigidly defined by formal status or routine, and activities tend to be more flexible and spontaneous. Rosengren and DeVault (1963) found that the formal relationships exhibited between physicians and nurses in a patient's room did not necessarily hold up when they moved out into the corridor. The corridor was the location where people could disagree, have doubts, or simply set their formal responsibilities aside and have casual conversations (Sommer, 1969). (In this behavioral sense, the staff lounge could also be considered an interstitial space.)

When a particular function is assigned to an interstitial space, it takes on several meanings or purposes (Fig. 16-3). It is a service space, a transitional zone, an edge between zones, and a very special place. It is also a tremendously complex design problem. It is exactly this attitude, however, which must be adopted if the birthing room is to become the central element in an environment for childbirth. It must be responsive to the needs of the frightened adolescent mother-to-be as well as the 30-year-old natural childbirth enthusiast. The birthing room zone can be characterized as interstitial space which separates the social and medical support zones, in which a mother or family can occupy and claim a particular module of space—a module which can be altered to suit the needs of the users. It

[2]The concept of articulated service space, or interstitial space, was created by Louis I. Kah in the A.N. Richardson Medical Research Laboratory project and the Salk Institute of Biological Studies Project.

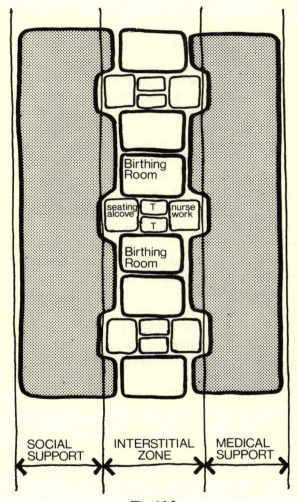

Fig. 16-3.

can be introverted or extroverted. It can open to the nurse station on one side, or the gallery and lounges on the other side. It can be a private space or a social space. It can offer the reassurance of all the potentially necessary emergency medical support, but not preclude the informality and comfort of a homelike environment (Fig. 16-4).

The individual birthing room environment is, therefore, the single most important space to be designed. The amount of space required is substantially more than would be required for a typical single bedroom because of the amount of services and furnishings necessary. Space is needed to allow the movement of medical staff and equipment. A private bathroom should be provided for each room, and storage is needed for personal belongings. A lounge with a chair or seating alcove provides a place to relax or get out of bed, and together with a small desk or counter adds to the residential quality of the space. This is also the area of the room which forms the link with the lounge or gallery areas in the social support zone. One should be able to open this area up to allow maximum social contact with family, or be able to close up that side and open the other side toward the nursing station area (Fig. 16-5).

All of the necessary medical support services (medical gases, monitoring equipment hookups, communication systems, electrical power) can be provided in the wall at the head of the bed (Fig. 16-6). If needed, everything is available even though most normal deliveries will not require such facilities. If surgical intervention is necessary, then the mother would have to be moved. The goal, however, is to have the healthiest baby possible in the most comfortable environment possible, and to give the mother more control of a wider range of options during childbirth.

SUMMARY AND CONCLUSIONS

The predominant issues in the design of environments for childbirth have shifted from "safety" and the "reduction of

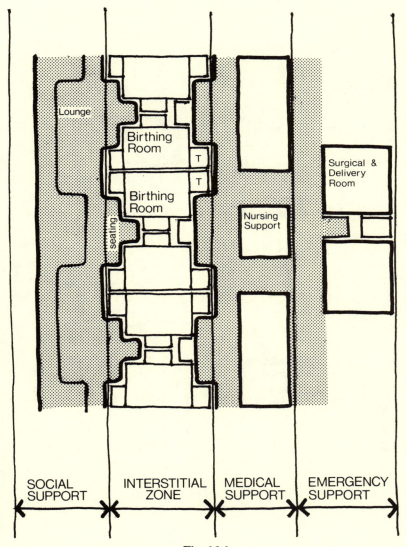

Lounge

Birthing
Room

T

T

Birthing
Room

seating

Nursing
Support

Surgical &
Delivery
Room

SOCIAL
SUPPORT

INTERSTITIAL
ZONE

MEDICAL
SUPPORT

EMERGENCY
SUPPORT

Fig. 16-4.

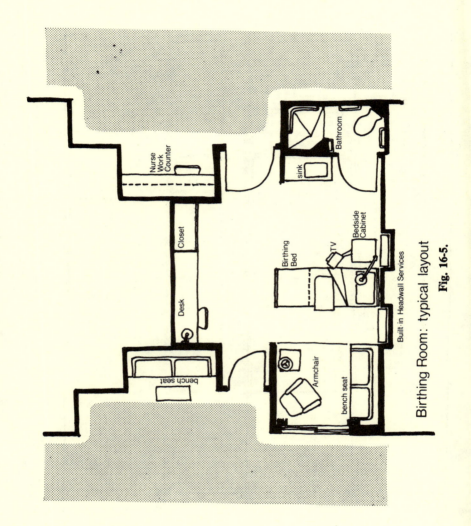

Birthing Room: typical layout

Fig. 16-5.

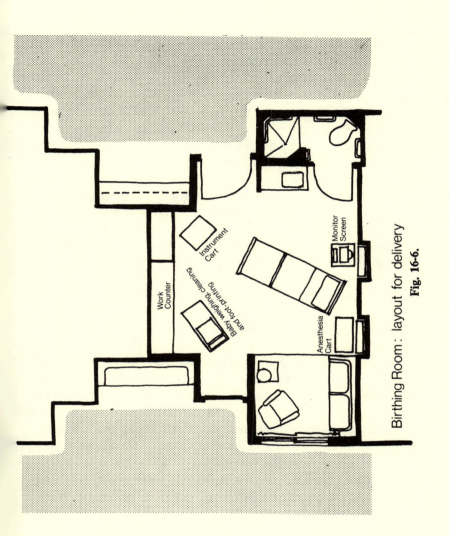

Birthing Room: layout for delivery

Fig. 16-6.

Monitor Screen

Instrument Cart

Work Counter

Baby weighing, cleaning and foot-printing

Anesthesia Cart

pain" to the provision of a wider range of options to a mother and/or family. The goal of a safe and healthy child has not taken a backseat, but it is recognized that several approaches are available for achieving that goal. The design of obstetrics and delivery facilities in the recent past has limited the options available to mothers because those designs have been based almost totally on functional criteria. Conversely, a total emphasis on social criteria could be just as limiting. A sensitive and responsive environment for childbirth requires an inclusive design methodology which structures the necessary compromises and elicits the compatible qualities from both functional and social design objectives.

Implicit with the provision of a wider range of options is the importance of providing additional social and psychological support for the mother. She must be better educated in the childbirth process and aware of her needs as well as the various methods available to meet those needs. The impact of these considerations on the design of the obstetrics and delivery department places the mother at the center of a range of environmental experiences. The birthing room becomes her own "personal space," her own territory which she can manipulate or adjust to satisfy her own needs and desires. The birthing room should be considered home base for the entire labor, delivery, and recovery process. She may opt to leave that room for either social or medical support, but she should always be able to reach back to its safety and security.

Finally, an overriding issue can be raised by the following questions: To what extent does the design of functionally specific environments in the community hospital foster a dependency on the health care provided in those environments and thereby reduce a patient's ability or desire to care for herself? And, how can the design of these environments help promote higher levels of individual competency in health care?

The issue of competency is important to all buildings designed for health care, but it is particularly important when considering childbirth environments because the vast majority of mothers will have normal, natural childbirths. They are not sick, and in the classic sense they should not be considered as patients receiving medical care. They are women going through the exciting, sometimes frightening, sometimes painful, and often physically exhausting experience of childbirth. They may need considerable support, both socially and medically, because it is a very unpredictable process. The design of an environment for childbirth must be responsive to all of these functional and social needs, and provide a quality of environment equal to the very special and extraordinary quality of the childbirth experience.

REFERENCES

Lubin, J. The birthing room: More hospitals offer maternity facilities that feel like home. *The Wall Street Journal,* Thursday, February 15, 1979.

Rosengren, W. & DeVault, S. The sociology of time and space in an obstetrical hospital. In Friedson, E. (Ed.). *The hospital in modern times.* New York: Free Press, 1963.

Sommer, R. *Personal space: The behavioral basis of design.* Englewood Cliffs, N.J.: Prentice-Hall, 1969.

Taylor, C. *In horizontal orbit: Hospitals and the cult of efficiency.* New York: Holt, 1970.

chapter 17

THE LEBOYER APPROACH
A New Concern for
the Psychological Aspects of
The Childbirth Experience

David Kliot
Louise Silverstein

The critical impact of pregnancy and childbirth on a woman's psychological organization has long been recognized in the literature (Anthony & Benedek, 1970; Bibring et al., 1961; Deutsch, 1948). In contrast, the manner in which the events of labor and delivery affect the infant's initial adaptive capacities and the process of early mother–infant bonding only recently have become issues of research interest (Eichler et al, 1977; Hutt, Lenard, Prechtl, 1969; Klaus & Kennell, 1974; Sugarman, 1976). Scientific interest is now being directed to whether certain obstetric procedures are more effective in stabilizing the infant's physiological equilibrium and in increasing his/her responsivity in reciprocal interactions. In addition, researchers are now exploring whether specific experiences associated with childbirth (e.g., immediate contact between mother and infant) generate more positive maternal attachment behaviors and thus enhance the process of maternal–infant adjustment.

The "Leboyer" method of childbirth management can be used as a vehicle for studying both of these issues. It is designed to minimize the physiological trauma of birth for the infant. Also it provides an opportunity for extended parent-infant contact immediately postpartum.

This chapter will describe the Leboyer approach to early newborn management. The preliminary research data available on the effect of this technique will be presented and the implications of these findings will be discussed in the context of recent research on infant postnatal adaptation and maternal–infant adjustment.

THE LEBOYER APPROACH TO EARLY NEWBORN CARE

Leboyer (1975), a French obstetrician, has argued against the efficacy of the entire system of traditional early newborn care. A standard pediatric textbook describes conventional delivery room management of the newborn as follows (Behrman, 1977):

> Immediately after delivery, the baby should be restrained with the head slightly dependent, while the cord is clamped and cut. The infant should then be placed supine on a table, the head kept low with a slight lateral tilt. A nurse should listen to the heartbeat immediately . . . the physician should aspirate the mouth, pharynx and nose with a catheter . . . lightly slapping the soles frequently aids in initiating a deep breath and crying. (p. 131)

> To diminish evaporative heat loss, the baby should be dried at once. Further heat loss . . . should be prevented by . . . placing the baby in an incubator, enclosing him in a silver swaddler or plastic bag, or providing a microenvironment of radiant heat over the resuscitation table. (p. 228)

Leboyer (1975) proposes that these "standard" procedures are not necessary for the physiological safety of the majority of healthy newborns and that they represent an invasive assault on the infant's sensibilities at a time of great vulnerability. He has developed an approach which purports to ease the transition from intra-to extrauterine life. Leboyer reduces the amount of auditory and visual stimulation with which the infant is initially bombarded. In order to maintain some aspects of the intrauterine environment, he delays uncurling the infant's spine and clamping the umbilical cord. He attempts to soothe the infant and restore some body heat by placing the neonate on the mother's abdomen and massaging its back. Then he returns the infant to a buoyant environment by bathing him or her in warm water for several minutes. Each procedure is designed to calm and soothe the infant in order to ease the immediate postnatal adaptation. The steps in a "Leboyer" delivery are outlined below.

Leboyer Method of Childbirth Management

1. Overhead lights are dimmed, delivery room door is closed, and staff maintains quiet.
2. As the infant is born, curvature of the spine is maintained, and the infant is placed face down on the mother's unprepped, undraped abdomen. The infant is gently massaged by the mother and/or obstetrician for 5 to 10 minutes. Nasopharyngeal suctioning is not done unless specific signs of respiratory distress are present.
3. The umbilical cord is not clamped and cut until it stops pulsating.
4. Then the infant is placed in a warm water (38° C) bath for approximately 5 minutes.

In contrast, in a standard delivery, the room is usually well-lighted and no effort is made to modify noise. The infant is held in either a head-dependent or supine position and its nose and mouth are suctioned. The umbilical cord is clamped within 60 seconds after birth, and the infant, if given to the mother, is swaddled and put on her draped abdomen. Frequently, the infant is immediately placed in an infant warmer.

Preliminary Research on the Effects of the LeBoyer Approach

Although Leboyer has delivered over 1000 infants using his technique, he has not systematically explored its effect on infant physiology and behavior. Because Leboyer's procedures represent radical departures from conventional management, it was important to demonstrate the safety of his approach. Kliot et al. (1979), studied the effect of a "modified Leboyer approach" (excluding the bath) on a wide range of physiological variables including heart rate, rectal temperature, hematocrit levels, blood pH, and bilirubin. They found that a sample of "Leboyer" infants (N=79) had physiological values within normal range values and equivalent to the values of a control group of 12 infants. Subsequent to this study, Kliot (1979) reports delivering over 1500 babies without complications using all of Leboyer's procedures. A modified technique utilizing postural drainage and the bath has also been incorporated in Cesarean section deliveries. These findings suggest that Leboyer's approach is physiologically safe for most healthy newborns.

Rapoport (1976) reports preliminary evidence to suggest that "the Leboyer experience" may favorably affect parental perceptions of their infants. In a retrospective study of 120 children, aged 1, 2, and 3 years, whose families had been assigned to Dr. Leboyer in a maternity clinic for delivery, Rapoport found that the parents described their "Leboyer" child as "easy," "delightful," and "unusually flexible." Multiparous mothers reported that their "Leboyer" child was much more adaptable than previous children. Only 10 of the 120 parents reported any developmental eating or sleeping difficulties. In addition, 100 percent of the mothers stated that they would choose this method of childbirth for the birth of their next child. These findings suggest that a "Leboyer" delivery experience may enhance parent–child adjustment and lessen the incidence of developmental psychosomatic disorders in childhood.

Other studies indicate that a Leboyer delivery is related to a decrease in the infant's internal physiological tension and to an increase in his/her alertness. Salter (1978) observed the state of six "Leboyer" and six control group infants during three 15-minute observation periods within the first 24 hours postpartum. Although she did not analyze her data statistically, she reports that the "Leboyer" infants spent more time in the quiet-alert state than did control group infants in all three observation periods. Oliver and Oliver (1978), observing spontaneous behaviors occuring in the delivery room during the first 15 minutes postpartum in "Leboyer" and control group infants (N=17 in each group), found that the "Leboyer" babies spent significantly ($p < .01$) more time with eyes open and hand muscles relaxed than did control group babies.

To summarize, although research on the effects of the Leboyer approach is still scanty and not rigorously designed, the preliminary findings suggest that this approach is physiologically safe and may be related to (1) a decrease in neonatal internal physiological tension, (2) an increase in alertness and responsivity to external stimulation and (3) a decrease in the incidence of developmental psychosomatic disorders.

RELATED RESEARCH ON INFANT POSTNATAL ADAPTATION AND MATERNAL–INFANT ATTACHMENT

Infant Postnatal Adaptation

If a Leboyer delivery succeeds in decreasing the trauma of birth for the infant, then he or she should become more accessible to external stimulation, and the process of active learning and reciprocal interaction with caretakers should be enhanced. The establishment of a stable internal equilibrium has been described as the major developmental task of the first 2 months of life (Emde & Robinson, 1976; Mahler, Pine, Bergman, 1975; Sander, 1969). However, relatively few researchers and clinicians have focused on the specific stresses which the birth process places on the infant's ability to establish that equilibrium.

Hutt, Lenard, and Prechtl (1969) have described this process of postnatal adaptation:

> The fetus lives relatively passively, in an environment with a constant temperature, regular oxygen supply and nutrition. Since it is suspended in amniotic fluid, it is not fully exposed to the force of gravity and sensory stimulation is weak. When, however, the infant is born, the conditions in which he lives change dramatically. With physical separation from the mother, he is exposed to a climatically, physiologically and nutritionally novel environment. This is a critical phase in the baby's development and carries great risks. He now has to work for food, regulate his own body temperature in a climatically inconstant environment, and breathe in order to secure oxygen. He is now fully exposed to gravity against which he must achieve at least rudimentary postural adjustments. Moreover, he is exposed to a whole range of novel sensory stimuli. (p. 130)

In addition to a general insensitivity to the stresses occasioned by the birth process, the scientific community traditionally has thought of the newborn infant as a relatively passive and undifferentiated organism who reacted to stimuli in a global and unorganized way. More recent information has shown the newborn to be active organism with definite stimulus needs, both for soothing and for arousal (Brazelton, 1973; Emde, Swedberg, Suzuki, 1975; Korner, 1969; Wolff, 1971).

Given this new understanding of the newborn infant's sensitivities, attention is now being directed to hospital procedures that may unnecessarily stress the infant's postnatal adaptation and subsequently interfere with early mother–infant bonding. Certain events of labor and delivery, such as length of labor and maternal medication are known to be important influences on the regulatory capacities of the infant (Aleksandrowicz & Aleksandrowicz, 1974; Emde & Koeni, 1969; Kron et al., 1966; Yang 1976). A recent trend has begun to question such hospital procedures as separation of mother and infant at birth and routine circumsion (Emde & Robinson, 1976; Klaus and Kennell, 1974; Sugarman, 1976).

The Leboyer approach is a part of this new trend in that it focuses on decreasing the stress of the entire transition from intrauterine to extrauterine life. Advocates of a "gentle birth" are responding to the relatively recent scientific awareness of the newborn infant as a sentient and sensitive being. If this technique can lessen the trauma of the immediate postnatal transition, the entire process of postpartum adaptation may be enhanced as well.

Maternal–Infant Attachment

The recognition of the infant as active and organized has generated a major research trend—studying the infant as part of an interactional system (Lewis & Rosenblum, 1974; Yarrow, 1974). Previously, researchers had been primarily concerned with the caregiver's role in nurturing and shaping infant behavior. Interaction was felt to be essentially unidirectional, going from mother to baby. More recently, mother and baby have come to be viewed as an interactional system in which each partner initiates and reinforces the behavior of the other. Thus, differences in infant responsivity are now understood to elicit differential caretaking.

Previous research indicated that the infant's ability to initiate interactions and to respond to maternal stimulation is a powerful influence on the mother's early feelings of attachment. Robson (1967) and Robson and Moss (1970) recognized the infant's role in eliciting positive attachment feelings. They found that mothers first reported feeling love for their infants when the baby appeared to be looking at them. Similarly, Thoman (1975) described how a rejecting baby, i.e., a baby who was awake and alert primarily while alone in bed and who became drowsy or fussy whenever picked up, could disrupt mother–infant synchrony.

Brazelton et al. (1975) and Stern (1974) have studied the manner in which newborn infants (aged 2 to 3 weeks) initiate and regulate mother–infant interaction. Stern (1974) found that mothers' speech patterns and facial expressions changed dramatically in response to infant gaze behavior. The infants were observed to have cyclical patterns of interaction which ranged from initiation of contact, to withdrawal from interaction. Mother–infant interaction sequences were successful only when the mother adapted to the infant's cues.

If the Leboyer approach to early newborn management enhances infant alertness and decreases irritability, infant responsivity to maternal stimulation and ability to elicit positive caretaking may be corresspondingly increased. Therefore, this childbirth approach may have an indirect, positive effect on mother–infant attachment. Leboyer's technique also may have a more direct impact on early bonding, because the procedures provide the mother (and father) an extended period of contact with the infant immediately postpartum. Some researchers (e.g., Klaus & Kennell, 1976) believe that the hour immediately postpartum is a critical period during which the process of maternal attachment can be either enhanced or disrupted. In a series of studies (deChateau & Wiberg, 1977 a, b; Hales et al., 1977; Kennell et al., 1974; Klaus et al., 1972) maternal behaviors and attitudes under varying conditions of extended early postpartum contact have been assessed.

An early Klaus-Kennell study (1974) examining the effect of 16 hours of extra contact throughout the hospital stay found differences in *en face* (holding the infant so that the mother's and infant's eyes are in the same vertical plane) and fondling behavior at one month postpartum. Mothers who had extra contact also reported less willingness to leave their infant and a greater tendency to pick the infant up during this first month. During pediatric examinations given at 1 month and 1 year, the extra contact group exhibited more proximity-maintaining and soothing behaviors than did the control group mothers.

Hales et al. (1977) provided three groups of mothers with variations in extended contact. One group had skin-to-skin contact in the first hour postpartum, another group had skin-to-skin contact for 45 minutes at 12 hours postpartum. The third group had no skin-to-skin contact. However, all mothers had some form of extended contact because, after 12 hours, the infants remained in the mothers' rooms throughout the hospital stay. At 36 hours postpartum, no differences were found between the 12-hour skin-to-skin group and the control group. However, the immediate postpartum skin-to-skin group differed from the other two groups in frequency of *en face* behavior.

deChateau and Wiberg (1977 a,b) provided an experimental group of primiparous mothers with 15 to 20 minutes of immediate skin-to-skin contact with their infants. Two routine care groups (primiparous and multiparous) received their clothed infants at 30 minutes postpartum either in their bed or next to their bed. All three groups remained with their infants for the next 2 hours. At 36 hours postpartum, deChateau found that the immediate skin-to-skin contact affected only mothers of boys. These mothers smiled at, burped, and held their infants more than did routine contact primiparous mothers of boys. At 3 months postpartum, the extra contact mothers of boys looked *en face* and kissed their infants more. Routine care primiparous mothers cleaned their girls more than did extra contact primiparous mothers of girls. The extra contact mothers reported breastfeeding longer and more easily adjusting to their child than did routine contact mothers. There were no significant differences between the extra contact mothers (all of whom were primiparous) and the routine contact multiparous group.

These studies suffer from major methodological limitations because the control group is not provided with an experience equivalent to that of the experimental group and failure to differentiate immediate skin-to-skin contact and extended contact throughout the hospital stay, etc. Taken as a whole, however, this body of research does indicate that extended early postpartum contact increases positive maternal attitudes and affectionate behaviors. Gaulin-Kraemer et al. (1977), in a more controlled study, lend support to this conclusion. In their study

28 mother–infant pairs with differing intervals of separation (10 to 25 hours before the first feeding) were observed. The sooner after delivery the first feeding occurred, the more the mother caressed her infant, talked to the infant, and held the infant before beginning the functional aspects of feeding.

The Leboyer approach must be considered within the context of the Klaus-Kennell research because it provides mother and infant with skin-to-skin contact immediately postpartum. Kliot (1979) has extended Leboyer's technique to a family-centered model by inviting the father to bathe the infant. Thus, mother-father-infant are afforded 20 to 30 minutes of early interaction. Other studies have shown that this kind of active participation in the events of labor and delivery improves the mother's evaluation of her delivery experience which in turn is related to positive early reactions to her infant (Davenport-Slack and Boylan, 1974; Doering & Entwisle, 1975; Newton & Newton, 1962; Steer, 1950).

In summary, variations in the management of labor, delivery, and the early postpartum period have been shown to be related to positive maternal attitudes and attachment behaviors. Because the Leboyer approach provides an opportunity for extended and active contact between mother and baby, this approach may enhance early mother–infant bonding.

CONCLUSION

The Leboyer approach to childbirth management is part of a current trend away from an emphasis on the medical mechanics of obstetric management and toward consideration of the effect of management techniques on the psychological well-being of mother and infant. Although only preliminary research evidence concerning the efficacy of this approach exists to date, certain conclusions can be drawn from the available data:

1. The Leboyer approach appears to be medically safe for the majority of healthy newborn infants.
2. The Leboyer approach is less invasive for the neonate than conventional obstetric procedures in terms of avoiding (a) nasopharyngeal suctioning, (b) auditory and visual overstimulation, (c) overt physical stimulation (e.g., slapping the soles of the feet) to initiate respiration. Since the Leboyer delivery is less invasive, the stress of the transition from intrauterine to extrauterine life may be decreased, and the process of postnatal adaptation correspondingly improved.
3. The Leboyer approach provides experiences that have been shown to increase positive maternal attachment behavior, e.g., active participation by both parents in the delivery experience and extended early mother–infant contact.

The medical community has historically been reluctant to utilize more psychologically-oriented approaches to childbirth such as family-centered childbirth, the use of midwives, and the Leboyer approach. This reluctance has been based, in part, on a concern for the physiological safety of patients. The recent research reviewed in this chapter indicates clearly, however, that the Leboyer approach is physiologically safe for most normal infants. This technique also provides both parents and infants with psychological experiences that are likely to have a positive effect on later adjustment. Thus, the Leboyer approach enables the concerned modern obstetrician to safeguard the psychological as well as the physiological needs of mother and child.

REFERENCES

Aleksandrowicz, M. K., & Aleksandrowicz, D. The effect of pain relieving drugs administered during labor and delivery on the behavior of the newborn. *Merrill Palmer Quarterly,* 1974, *20,* 121–141.

Anthony, E. J., & Benedek, T., *Parenthood: it's psychology and psychopathology.* Boston: Little, Brown, 1970.

Behrman, R. E. (Ed.). *Neonatal-perinatal medicine,* 2nd Ed. St. Louis: Mosby, 1977.

Bibring, G., Dwyer, T. F., Huntington, D. S., Valenstein, A. F. A study of the psychological processes in pregnancy and of the earliest mother-child relationship. *Psychoanalytic Study of the Child,* 1961, *16,* 9–72.

Brazelton, T. B. *Neonatal behavioral assessment scale.* Spastics International Medical Publication. London: William Heinemann, 1973.

Brazelton, T. B., Tronick, E., Adamson, L., Als, H., & Wise, S. Early mother-infant reciprocity; In *Parent-infant interaction, Ciba Foundation Symposium* 33. Amsterdam: Elsevier; 1975.

Davenport-Slack, B., & Boylan, C. H., Psychological correlates of childbirth pain. *Psychosomatic Medicine,* 1974, *36,* 215–223.

deChateau, P., & Wiberg, B. Long-term effect on mother-infant behaviors of extra contact during the first hour postpartum. I. First observations at 36 hours. *Acta Paediatrica Scandinavica,* 1977a, *66,* 137–144.

deChateau, P., & Wiberg, B. Long-term effect on mother-infant behaviors of extra contact during the first hour postpartum. II. A follow-up at three months. *Acta Paediatrica Scandinavica,* 1977b, *66,* 144–151.

Deutsch, H. *The psychology of women,* vol. 2. New York: Grune & Stratton, 1945.

Doering, S. G., & Entwisle, D. R. Preparation during pregnancy and ability to cope with labor and delivery. *American Journal of Orthopsychiatry,* 1975, *44,* 825–829.

Eichler, L. S., Winickoff, S. A., Grossman, F. K., Ansalone, M. K., & Grofseyeff, M. H. Adaptation to pregnancy, birth and early parenting: a preliminary view. Paper presented at the meeting of the American Psychological Association, San Francisco, August, 1977.

Emde, R. N., & Koenig, K. Neonatal smiling, frowning and rapid eye movement states, II. Sleep-cycle study. *Journal of the American Academy of Child Psychiatry,* 1969, *8,* 637–656.

Emde, R. N., & Robinson, J. The first two months: recent research in developmental psychology and the changing view of the newborn; In J. Noshpitz & J. Call (Eds.). *Basic Handbook of Child Psychiatry.* New York: Basic Books, 1976.

Emde, R. N., Swedberg, J., & Suzuki, B. Human wakefulness and biological rhythms after birth. *Archives of General Psychiatry,* 1975, *32,* 780–783.

Gaulin-Kraemer, E., Shaw, J. L., & Thoman, E. B. Mother-infant interaction at first prolonged encounter: Effects of variation in delay after delivery. Paper presented at the meeting of the Society for Research in Child Development, New Orleans, March, 1977.

Hales, D. J., Lozoff, B., Sosa, R., & Kennell, J. H. Defining the limits of the maternal sensitive period. *Developmental Medicine and Child Neurology,* 1977, *19,* 454–461.

Hutt, S. J. Lenard, H. G., & Prechtl, H. F. R. Psycho-physiological studies in newborn infants. In L. Lipsett & H. Reese (Eds.). *Advances in Child Development and Behavior,* vol. 4. New York: Academic Press, 1969.

Kennell, J. H., Jerauld, R., Wolfe, H. Chesler, D., Kreger, N. C., McAlpine, W., Steffa, M., & Klaus, M. H. Maternal behavior one year after early and extended post-partum contact. *Developmental Medicine and Child Neurology,* 1974, *16,* 172–179.

Klaus, M. H., Jerauld, R., Kreger, N. C., McAlpine, W., Steffa, M. & Kennell, J. H. Maternal attachment: importance of the first post-partum days. *New England Journal of Medicine,* 1972, *286,* 460–463.

Klaus, M. H., & Kennell, J. H., *Maternal-infant bonding.* St. Louis: Mosby, 1976.

Kloit, D., Personal communication, January 1979.

Kliot, D., Lilling, M., Silverstein, L., & Fisher, B. Changing maternal/newborn care: an empirical study of the Leboyer approach to childbirth management. Manuscript submitted for publication, March, 1979.

Korner, A. Neonate startles, smiles, erections and reflex sucks as related to state, sex and individuality. *Child Development,* 1969, *40,* 1039–1053.

Kron, R. E., Stein, M., & Goddard, K. R. Newborn sucking behavior affected by obstetric sedation. *Pediatrics,* 1966, *37,* 1012–1016.

Leboyer, F., *Birth, without violence.* New York: Knopf, 1975.

Lewis, M., & Rosenblum, L., *The effect of the infant on its caregiver.* New York: Wiley, 1974.

Mahler, M., Pine, F., & Bergman, A. *The psychological birth of the human infant.* New York: Basic Books, 1975.

Newton, N., & Newton, M. Mothers' reactions to their newborn babies. *Journal of the American Medical Association,* 1962 *181,* 206–210.

Oliver, C. M., & Oliver, G. M., Gentle birth: its safety and its effect on neonatal behavior. *Journal of Obstetrics, Gynecology and Neonatal Nursing,* 1978, *5,* 35–40.

Rapoport, D. Pour une naissance sans violence: resultats d'une premiere enquete. *Bulletin de Psychologie,* 29, 1976, *322,* 552–560.

Robson, K. The role of eye to eye contact in maternal-infant attachment. *Journal of Child Psychology and Psychiatry,* 1967, *8,* 13–25.

Robson, K. S., & Moss, H. A. Patterns and determinants of maternal attachment. *Journal of Pediatrics,* 1970, *77,* 976–985.

Salter, A. Birth without violence: a medical controversy. *Nursing Research,* 1978, *27,* 84–88.

Sander, L. Regulation and organization in the early infant-caretaker system.

In R. Robinson (Ed.). *Brain and early behavior.* London: Academic Press, 1969.

Steer, C. M., The effect of type of delivery on future childbearing. *American Journal of Obstetrics and Gynecology,* 1950, *60,* 395–400.

Stern, D. N. Mother and infant at play: the dyadic interaction involving facial, vocal and gaze behavior; In M. Lewis & L. Rosenblum (Eds.). *The effect of the infant on its caregiver.* New York: Wiley, 1974.

Sugarman, M. Paranatal influences on maternal attachments. *American Journal of Orthopsychiatry,* 1977, *47,* 17–31.

Thoman, E. How a rejecting baby may affect mother-infant synchrony; In *Parent-infant interaction, Ciba Foundation Symposium 33.* Amsterdam: Elsevier, 1975.

Wolff, P. Organization of behavior in the first three months of life; In J. I. Nurnberger (Ed.). *Biological and Environmental Determinants of Early Development.* Baltimore: Williams & Wilkins, 1971.

Yang, R. K., Zweig, A. R., Douthitt, T. C., & Federman, E. J. Successive relationships between maternal attitudes during pregnancy, analgesic medication during labor and delivery, and newborn behavior. *Developmental Psychology,* 1976, *12,* 6–14.

Yarrow, L. J. Parents and infants: an interactive network. Paper presented at the meeting of the American Psychological Association, New Orleans, August, 1974.

chapter 18

THE BIRTH OF AN ABNORMAL CHILD

Alan R. Fleischman, Donna Sands Fryd

Changes in societal norms and advances in medical technology have combined to make the birth of an abnormal child in modern-day America an even more devastating event today than it was just a few years ago. Families in all socioeconomic classes have changed greatly in recent years. The incidence of extended or multiple generation families is decreasing. Thus, the loving grandmother or elderly aunt who could care for the abnormal infant and support the family through this crisis is not available. Furthermore, with the diminishing birth rate due to planned parenthood and birth control, family size is limited. In the past, in large families, there was room for a child who was slow or abnormal. He could blend in with the larger whole of the family. Today, with fewer children being conceived, women are expecting a good product of their pregnancy. Medical advances, research, and lay literature support these expectations. Women believe that adequate prenatal care and concern for one's nutrition and medical needs during pregnancy, combined with the new techniques of prenatal diagnosis, will likely result in a normal pregnancy and child. Furthermore, with the advances in fetal monitoring during labor and newborn care, it is anticipated that newborns will not only survive the birth process but will do well with no residual damage. In reality, although obstetric care, antenatal diagnosis, and neonatal medicine have dramatically affected survival rate and morbidity statistics over the last 20 years, there is still a significant number of neonates born prematurely or with a congenital anomaly or with significant disease.

Along with the advances in the field of perinatal medicine has come increasing concern about the ethics of the perinatal period. Professionals and lay people alike are concerned about the ethical issues related to pregnancy and childbirth such as abortion, age, and size of fetal viability and the maintenance through heroic measures of babies who are either neurologically impaired or have a significant congenital anomaly. However, little is written in the lay or professional literature about the psychological devastation created by the birth of an abnormal child. This chapter will first briefly overview the psychology of pregnancy as attitudes and feelings toward and during pregnancy affect attitudes to the newborn. Then, with the aid of case illustrations, the feelings related to the birth of a normal and abnormal child will be explored and some practical guidelines for the professional care of families in crisis will be proposed.

THE PSYCHOLOGY OF PREGNANCY

The prior psychological makeup of both mother and father, their relationship to each other, their interaction with significant others, and numerous social and economic considerations determine the psychological adaptation of the couple to the decision to have a child and to the events of the subsequent pregnancy. The decision to become pregnant need not always be a conscious one and may, in fact, have little to do with the actual desire to be pregnant or to have a child. The desire to prove sexual adequacy, normalcy, and health, as well as expressions of anger, rebellion, or depression may be part of the initial decision to become pregnant. Furthermore, the desire to produce someone to love and to be loved by is often a major motivating factor. Pregnancies are frequently perceived as a method of saving or solidifying a marriage in which the participants are having problems. The addition of a child as the focus for the father and mother may be a method of getting around the actual problem of interacting between the two participants. Defining and understanding, even retrospectively, the feelings about the decision to become pregnant aid in the evaluation of the feelings about the pregnancy and the newborn infant. If the decision to become pregnant was never made or was unclear, then the feelings around the decision to remain pregnant must be explored. The support of both partners is necessary to allow for good initial adaptation to the pregnancy. The woman must come to grips with the reality of the major changes that will occur in herself and her life and the long-term responsibilities and commitments consistent with the decision to be pregnant and to remain pregnant.

In the first weeks and months of pregnancy, the woman may deny the reality of the event. Actual changes in her physical being are minimal and there may be no change in her life-style. However, most women are aware that they are pregnant on a physical as well as an emotional level. The physical symptoms of nausea, gastrointestinal discomfort, changes in breasts, and body habitus may be exaggerated by the woman in conflict about her pregnancy. This is a time of great need for the pregnant woman. She requires the reassurance of her partner, the support of her friends and relatives, and medical support to assure the normalcy of herself and her pregnancy. At this stage in pregnancy, women do not focus on the reality of "having a child," but rather are more concerned about "being pregnant." Discussion of these initial feelings about the pregnancy, the changes in husband/wife relations, the feelings about sexuality and anticipatory feelings about motherhood can be extremely helpful in understanding the response to the newborn infant.

As the pregnancy continues into the fourth and fifth months, the reality of the fetus and its relationship to the mother becomes primary. The physical changes in the woman's body, combined with the movement of the fetus in utero, are a constant reminder of the pregnancy.

With the growth of her abdomen, the pregnant woman begins to relate to her fetus. She often decides on its sex, gives it a nickname, and begins to fantasize about the child's role in the family. Women frequently relate during this period to their own experiences in childhood. They begin to anticipate the need to be a mother and verbalize the desire either to duplicate the activities of their own nurturing mother or to be quite different. Most begin to read about motherhood and child care and manifest an interest in the furniture and clothing for the new child. The woman who is in conflict about her pregnancy at this point often sublimates or represses these feelings. These middle months of pregnancy are often associated with a decrease in the incidence of nausea, gastrointestinal discomfort, and fatigue which allows the mother to have a more positive attitude about the pregnancy and the impending delivery. A euphoric sense often occurs which may mask many of the fears and concerns of the pregnant woman. Men, too, become more aware of their unborn child and begin to anticipate with both joy and apprehension their new roles as fathers. The entire family begins to give increasing attention to the fetus. This developmental process of maternal-paternal-fetal relationship is important in determining the feelings toward the newborn.

As the end of pregnancy approaches, the euphoria and inner peace associated with the developing fetus gives way to an increasing anxiety about the imminence of the delivery. Parents become concerned about their ability to care for their child and often express the desire to be good parents. In addition, they become increasingly fearful that their child will not be normal. This can often be a time of great strain between the parents, each not wishing to verbalize his or her concerns in order to protect the other. As the last weeks of pregnancy approach, there is a desire to end the process and to have the reality of the birth occur. The anticipation and excitement are tremendous, but the discomforts, anxieties, and fears usually outweigh the positive feelings. During this period sexual interaction between mother and father often cease. This heightens the anxiety between them and many times causes the male partner to seek alternative methods of gratification. The feelings manifested toward the end of pregnancy, and the parents' ability to cope, are the direct precursors of the feelings that will be manifested at the time of the birth of the baby. Even the most sophisticated parents may have been frightened by and felt guilty for the multiple, ambivalent feelings they experienced during the pregnancy. Thus, exploration of these feelings is of great importance when discussing the birth of the child. A thorough examination of the feelings about pregnancy by the parents of a newborn child will greatly enhance the understanding of their response to the baby.

The Birth of the Child

The actual birth of the baby is often an anticlimax to the family. Just as the anticipation of a gift is often greater than the reality, the birth of the child is often a letdown. Disappointment, fear, anger, and depression sometimes are associated with the actual delivery of the baby. Both mother and father now must face the subliminal fears of inadequacy and inability to care for the new human being. Concerns about financial matters may become evident. The mother may now have to give up a money-making job, and the father is concerned about the adequacy of his ability to support his new family. Furthermore, this new person in the family may be viewed as a potential intrusion on the intimacy and closeness of the two parents.

On the other hand, the birth of a normal child reaffirms the parents' belief in their normalcy and culminates the excitement at the capability of creating a person in one's own image. There is great relief that the child appears to be normal. There is, however, a great need for this observation to be confirmed. The physician and nurse caring for the infant can aid the family with appropriate support and concern. The realization must be made that this newborn is special to its parents, even though it is a "routine well baby" to the nursery staff. Any minor deviation from normal is exaggerated by the parent, and these concerns should not be ignored by the professional. Explanations and clear answers to questions, along with anticipatory guidance, are indicated.

For the parent whose child is identified as potentially sick or abnormal a difficult time begins. The newborn infant is initially felt by his parents to be an extension of themselves. Therefore, if there is anything wrong, their feelings of worth and self-esteem are greatly affected. All the parents' earlier fears that their child would not be normal are reactivated and confirmed. The joy that is often associated with an infant's birth is diminished and the parents may feel a sense of fear, failure, guilt, anger, or depression. Although each family will react to this crisis in their own way, we have found that there are common themes and feelings which surround the birth of an abnormal child. Actual cases help to point out some of the feelings that are aroused by the birth of an abnormal child and to illustrate how families can be helped to adjust to this crisis.

L. was the second child of the A. family who was admitted to the Special Care Nursery shortly after birth because of jaundice, possibly due to an infection. Mr. and Mrs. A. had waited for 6 years before having their second child. They were anxiously anticipating the birth of this baby and had no reason to expect that this child would be less healthy than their first child. Although Mr. and Mrs. A. were quite happy about the pregnancy, this happiness was marred by the fact that shortly before L.'s birth, Mr. A. had been laid off from his job. Mr. A.'s general feeling of self-esteem and adequacy was threatened by this change. Although the family seemed to be coping with this financial problem fairly well, there was little doubt that they were under considerable stress.

L.'s condition was explained to Mr. and Mrs. A., and they were encouraged to visit with her. Mr. and Mrs. A. were unable to comprehend what was wrong with their baby. They were terrified by the noise and special equipment of the Special Care Nursery and felt generally overwhelmed and confused. While Mrs. A. was anxious and expressed feelings of fear and depression, Mr. A. acted angry and suspicious. He seemed unable to believe the doctors and occasionally blamed them for creating his baby's illness.

Throughout the first few days of L.'s life, Mr. and Mrs. A. needed repeated explanations regarding the cause of their daughter's problems and the recommended treatment plan. Mr. A. was rather demanding, anxious, and highly sensitive. Technical terms served to confuse and terrify the family while explanations that were too simplistic caused them to feel infantalized and ridiculed. The family's anger and anxiety were heightened when blood cultures revealed that the baby had a serious infection and that additional antibiotic therapy was needed. Additional meetings were held with L.'s parents, her doctor, and a social worker. L.'s condition and entire hospital course were again described to Mr. and Mrs. A. They were helped to express their fears and anxieties and were reassured about both their own reactions and L.'s progress and prognosis. Gradually the A.'s were able to calm down and feel less angry, threatened, and overwhelmed. The child did well and was discharged home in good condition.

The birth of a small, premature infant also produces a crisis for the family. Many of the same feelings are aroused, but these feelings are manifested in a somewhat different way.

T. was Ms. C.'s first child. She was born prematurely at 28 weeks gestation and 1050 grams (2 pounds, 5 ounces) and required 3 months of hospitalization. While hospitalized she suffered from respiratory difficulties, jaundice, and required blood transfusions.

Ms. C. visited T. within the first 24 hours of her life. She spoke with her daughter's doctors and nurses. Ms. C. was initially unable to cope with the situation. She was extremely concerned about her baby but was terrified. Ms. C. was astonished by the size and appearance of T. and felt that she did not really look like a baby. She feared that her child might not survive and asked many questions regarding the causes of T.'s premature birth. Ms. C. feared that a previous abortion or the fact that she did not severely restrict her activities during her pregnancy had caused T.'s premature birth. Ms. C. also felt guilty because she was somewhat repulsed by her daughter's appearance and because she still felt unprepared for motherhood.

Ms. C. initially found it very difficult to visit T. She felt somewhat helpless and continued to fear that T. might die. Gradually she began to overcome her shock and fear and became attached to T. At the same time, however, she expressed feelings of failure and a loss of self-esteem because she had been unable to carry her baby full term. Ms. C. also began to focus on her fears regarding her ability to be a good mother. She began to finish the preparations for motherhood that generally occur during the final months of the pregnancy. She thought about her own childhood, the early loss of her mother, and the nurturing that she later received from her stepmother. Ms. C. began to prepare emotionally and physically for her baby's homecoming. She became increasingly concerned about T.'s future development.

T.'s father was not living with the family. He found it difficult to visit T. and visited rather infrequently. He tried to support Ms. C., although he apparently found it difficult to deal with her anxiety. T.'s father was able to become more attached to her after she was discharged from the hospital.

The birth of a genetically abnormal infant is often devastating to the family.

J. was Mr. and Mrs. B.'s second child. Mrs. B. had been pregnant a number of times since the birth of her first child 9 years before. Each prior pregnancy had ended in a miscarriage. The B.'s were therefore quite nervous throughout the pregnancy. Their anxiety was heightened when Mrs. B. was advised, because of her age of 37, to undergo an amniocentesis. Two attempts to obtain amniotic fluid were unsuccessful and the family decided not to have any additional tests performed. They began to prepare for the birth and prayed that their unborn child would be normal. When J. was born after a 9-month gestational period, Mr. and Mrs. B. were overjoyed. Their joy was short-lived, however, because within 24 hours they were told that their infant appeared to have Down's syndrome. J. also had congenital heart disease and mild heart failure. She needed special formula, medications, and will eventually require heart surgery.

Mrs. B. expressed shock, disappointment, anger, and guilt. Both Mr. and Mrs. B. seemed to use denial. Mr. B. tended to treat J. normally and seemed to "forget" her diagnosis. Mrs. B., on the other hand, never forgot that her daughter was special, although she tended to attribute her specialness to her heart defect rather than to the fact that she had Down's syndrome.

Both Mr. and Mrs. B. searched for a reason for J.'s problem. They tended to blame themselves and each other. Mrs. B., once a religious woman, lost her faith. She was angry with God, herself, and J. Mr. B. spent more and more time away from home, working overtime, and drinking. The extended family refused to treat J. with the same love and attention that other babies in the family received. The family warned Mrs. B. that J. was going to die. Mrs. B. reacted to this and to her own feelings of guilt and anger by becoming overinvolved with J. She evidenced depression and a mourning reaction and found that she was preoccupied, anxious, and short-tempered. J.'s older sister, too, had great difficulty adjusting to her younger, "special" sister. It seems that this child would have had some problems even if her sister were normal, but J.'s specialness and Mrs. B.'s overinvolvement and high level of anxiety made the adjustment particularly hard for this child. J's sister began to misbehave at home, performed poorly in school, and generally evidenced infantile, regressive behavior.

For months following J.'s birth, she, her older sister, and Mrs. B. were seen frequently by the family's pediatrician and a social worker. Repeated attempts to meet and speak with Mr. B. were unsuccessful. The family needed continuing help in interpreting and understanding all aspects of J.'s condition. They also needed assistance in uncovering and understanding their ambivalent and angry feelings about J. Gradually Mrs. B. came to a fuller understanding and acceptance of J.'s problems. The family gained additional assistance as they became involved in a special program for infants with Down's syndrome and their families. The family will need continued support and assistance for a long time.

A devastating event in any family is the birth of a severely asphyxiated, brain-damaged newborn. The kinds of feelings are again similar, but emphasis is different.

M. was the first child for this young couple. M.'s mother had a very difficult time during her labor and delivery. She was so uncooperative that the obstetric staff was unable to use fetal monitoring to assess progress of labor. M. suffered severe perinatal asphyxia and was severely neurologically impaired at birth. M.'s critical condition and poor prognosis were explained to his parents and grandparents. The family was encouraged to visit and touch their baby. Pediatricians, nurses, and a social worker met with the family repeatedly to explain their infant's condition and to help them express their feelings and questions.

The family's initial reactions included feelings of blame, guilt, denial, anger, shock, and depression. M.'s parents and extended family members were extremely angry at the obstetric staff and blamed the obstetricians and nurse midwives for M.'s severe damage. Angry with M.'s mother for other reasons, some members of the family implied that M.'s problems were caused by his mother having cared for herself inadequately during the pregnancy.

At times, the family used both denial and fantasy. They talked about their infant as if he would survive and be perfectly normal. At other times they would express their commitment to this child no matter how severely damaged he was. These feelings were periodically interrupted by a true and complete understanding of M.'s problems. At such times, M.'s parents would become somewhat overwhelmed with feelings of grief and depression. M. died a few days after his birth. His parents and family members were not terribly surprised by his death, although their fantasies and hopes had continued throughout his short life. With M.'s death, the entire family began to truly mourn their loss. Approximately 6 weeks after M.'s death, family members returned to the hospital to speak with M.'s doctors and social worker. M.'s problems were discussed and the family's questions were answered. The family seemed to be adapting well to the loss and required no ongoing counseling or referral.

PRACTICAL GUIDELINES

Parental feelings aroused by the birth of the normal and abnormal child differ only in intensity and emphasis. Denial, fear, anger, depression, elation, and guilt combine to form the framework of the parents' emotions. Understanding and exploring these feelings allow the professional to help the family cope with this life crisis.

Operationally, how does this process work? First, the pediatrician responsible for a newborn's care should meet the family for a prenatal visit. The goals of this visit include sharing ideas about nutrition and care for the newborn and helping the parents to anticipate the needs of the new child. This visit is a concrete statement that the parents do not deny the child. It allows the pediatrician and family to begin to develop a relationship which will be built upon after the birth of the child. This visit is of great importance particularly if a problem arises in the newborn period.

Next, the obstetrician or midwife delivering the infant must be open and honest about the condition of the fetus and newborn. If there are reasons to be concerned during labor, the parents should at least have some understanding of the problem. A sudden fetal demise or delivery of an asphyxiated newborn will require all the strength the family can muster. This is usually best coped with if there is some time to digest and understand what has transpired.

With the birth of a child, the professional examining the infant should be clear in relating his observations to the parents. If there is a question or problem, he should be honest about his concerns. With a specifically abnormal child, we believe that the family should be informed on the first day of life about what is known concerning the child's condition. We often see the mother of a sick neonate in the obstetric recovery area to report to her on the condition of her few-hour-old infant. This is followed by a visit to her hospital room 6 to 8 hours later for further explanation and clarification and an invitation to visit the sick newborn. It is important that the pediatrician and obstetrician communicate with each other and do not give different messages to the parents or use the neonate as a vehicle to express hostility between themselves.

Hospital practices can enhance the relationship between parents and newborns, even in the care of an abnormal infant. A neonatal intensive care unit should encourage family visits and participation in newborn care. Even the sickest infant can be touched by the parents. We believe that pathologic grief can be decreased by the attachment of the family to the infant, even if he will eventually die.

At approximately 3 days of age the physician, social worker, and nurse caring for the infant should formally meet with the parents. This session is used to explain again what is known about the illness, the plan for medical care, and prognosis. The family is encouraged to ask questions and share concerns on their own level and as they perceive them. The professionals can explore what problems exist for the family. The mother is about to go home without her infant. What are her feelings about this? Is there a grandmother or significant other relative whose reaction is of particular concern to the parents? Would it be helpful for the social worker or physician to speak to these people? What will the parents tell their family about this illness? What supports do they have at home?

As the child's condition changes, the family should be encouraged to continue a close relationship to the staff in the nursery and to the newborn infant. As soon as possible, parents are encouraged to participate in the care of their baby. Frequent visits and phone calls are important. We monitor these carefully and initiate calls to any family who seems reluctant or distant.

Each family will react to the birth of an abnormal child differently. In general, however, families are initially overwhelmed and are unable to comprehend the information they are being given. They are unable to think of all their questions and are frightened of verbalizing their fears. Sensitive listening to and recognition of the parents' underlying anxieties is of great assistance. Explaining common reactions and assuring parents that their reactions are not unusual can often be quite beneficial. Helping parents to express, recognize, and work through their guilt, anger, and ambivalent feelings is also indicated.

As mentioned previously, the intensity and duration of the crisis will depend on the infant's condition, the parents' understanding of it, their prior psychological state, and their reactions to the pregnancy. The family's need for continuing counseling will depend on their reaction to the crisis. Some families find it too painful and threatening to discuss their thoughts and feelings after the initial crisis or prefer to share such things only with close family members. The wishes of such families must be respected unless there is reason to suspect that they are unable to become attached to their babies. Other families need to be seen on a regular basis. This crisis may give them the opportunity to work through previous unresolved conflicts. Sometimes the birth of an abnormal child tends to exacerbate preexisting marital discord. On other occasions, parents who have different styles of coping are unable to understand their partner and new arguments ensue. Ongoing counseling with parents should involve helping them deal with these issues. Families will also need assistance in dealing with the questions and reactions of other family members and friends. Siblings of the sick newborn must also be helped. Helping parents to anticipate and prepare for questions and reactions is of invaluable assistance to everyone involved.

Throughout the infant's hospitalization, hospital routines, medical procedures, and information regarding the baby's condition must be explained to families. Families should be encouraged to ask questions and assured that no question is too small or insignificant. Complete understanding and acceptance of a baby's condition usually require much repetition. Gradually, as the baby improves, parents will be able to direct their attention away from their own feelings and will be able to focus on the future needs of their infant. Some parents will need time and help in finishing the preparations for parenthood that were interrupted by the birth of their premature infants. Other parents will need help in accomplishing the tasks involved in mourning the loss of their perfect child and accepting and becoming attached to their infant. Parents often fantasize and fear that their child will be permanently damaged. Some infants will, in fact, have special needs, while others will be fine. Parents must be given realistic and truthful answers to their questions. When there is no reason to expect that the baby will have additional difficulties, parents should be helped to work through all their feelings so that they can accept this child without making him too special. If, on the other hand, the child can be expected to suffer from continuing problems, the family needs help in understanding and accepting the needs of their special child. If the family has begun to work through their ambivalent feelings about their baby and if they have a good understanding of what they can expect in the future, they will be more willing and able to accept referrals to outside agencies for additional assistance. Referrals may include agencies for special medical needs, for infant stimulation programs, or for continuing psychological counseling.

The birth of a baby is an event which usually results in a family response of joy and happiness. However, the birth of an abnormal newborn is a crisis with the possibility of devastating consequences. Concerned, coordinated, compassionate care by professionals can greatly aid in the adaptation of the family to the birth of an abnormal child.

chapter 19

EFFECTS AND IMPLICATIONS OF A STILLBIRTH OR OTHER PERINATAL DEATH

Hazelanne Lewis

This century has seen changes in many of the mores of our society. What previously was unacceptable is now accepted openly. Medical scientists have succeeded in finding cures for many of what used to be fatal illnesses. Parents have fewer children and expect them to be born alive and well. Death is removed from the everyday life of young people and frequently only in their middle age do they have to deal with it. New taboos have sprung up about death, and less time has been allowed to mourn those who have died. When one takes these factors into account, it is possible to understand why stillbirths are rarely mentioned in anything other than medical textbooks. These texts usually confine themselves to causes and do not examine emotional effects. With both medical and social scientists experiencing difficulty in looking at the effects of stillbirth on families, it is not surprising that parents have difficulty in contemplating its possibility. To anticipate death in one's body while it is nourishing and bringing forth life is unthinkable.

Thus a stillbirth, when it occurs, is a shock and usually something outside the experience of the parents and their family.

After any death, the bereaved go through a period of mourning. This is also true after a stillbirth. However, the special circumstances surrounding a stillbirth make it difficult for mourning to be completed. This can lead to difficulties for the family with undue stress being placed on existing or subsequent children. To enable adequate help to be offered to these families, it is necessary to look at the events around a stillbirth in order to see what these problems are, how they arise, and to examine ways of avoiding them. Help can be offered to bereaved parents on an individual or on a group basis.

Many pregnant women have fears about whether their babies will be healthy and normal. Some are able to contemplate giving birth to a premature child and to imagine the anxiety that they would have at such a time. Few, unless they have had prior contact with stillbirths, are able to envisage a situation where their baby will die inside them. Because of this difficulty in anticipating death while pregnant, it is often difficult for women to accept the possibility that their baby may die. Thus, complications that arise in pregnancy may be understood after an explanation, but the implications for their baby can be suppressed and denied.

> A 34-year-old woman had married late. Both she and her husband had needed medical treatment in order to become fertile. While pregnant, she remained at work for as long as she could. When she attended for her 28 week antenatal checkup, it was discovered that her blood pressure was too high. She was admitted straight from the clinic to the antenatal ward, where she stayed for 5 weeks. Throughout this time, she remained hypertensive. The baby's progress was monitored regularly and the doctors expressed their concern for the baby to her. Unable to contemplate anything happening to the baby, she interpreted this as concern for her. As she did not feel ill, she was restless and resentful. Eventually, at 33 weeks, a cesarean section was performed in an attempt to save the baby's life. Unfortunately, the

baby died soon after birth while the mother was still under sedation. When seen 4 weeks later, she was resentful, bitter, and untrusting towards her doctors. She saw them as having killed her baby in order to maintain her health. When told that the cesarean section has been performed to save the baby's life, she was shocked. No one had bluntly said that her baby would die inside her if it was not removed. The words used had been "We are concerned about the baby, so we are going to take it out." Her denial had suppressed the meaning of these words. This new view of the reason for the birth/death of her baby brought different problems to adjust to, but enabled her to contemplate another baby as she now had more trust in the medical profession.

This ability to deny the possibility of their baby's death makes it difficult to care for mothers where there is a problem in their pregnancy. Undue pessimism can also cause problems. However, most parents prefer to be told the facts simply. Their denial can then leave them the choice of not asking the questions that will make them face reality. A lot of resentment is expressed when one parent is told of probable difficulties and then advised not to worry the other parent about it.

If the baby dies in utero, the mother has the horror of walking around with a dead baby inside her. One of the taboos that death carries in our society results in corpses being viewed with horror. To have a dead baby inside you is to be a contaminated person. Mothers feel unclean and some cannot bear to be touched. Despite rational knowledge to the contrary, some fear that they may die during labor as they are "walking death."

It was 4 days from the time my baby died until it was born. I spent the time alternating between being calm (especially when my children came to see me) and rushing out crying hysterically into the corridor. I was convinced that I too would die in labor as a punishment for allowing my baby to die. Labor was like all my births, quick and easy. Even after the baby was delivered I still expected to haemorrhage and die.

Obstetricians are reluctant to induce labor as soon as the baby dies because of complications that can arise if the induction is not successful. They are reluctant to have to submit the mother to an unnecessary cesarean section although many mothers plead for one in an attempt to tear the death from their body. It is difficult to strike the balance between medical and emotional priorities, but it should be noted that mothers who are left too long with a dead baby inside them may have difficulty in completing their mourning later. As with all deaths, it is hard to accept that the baby is dead. The mother remains overtly pregnant and it is not possible to verify the baby's death by visual or tactile means.

> It was 5 days from the time we were told that the baby was dead until labor started. We used to take turns to cry. First my husband would cry and I would comfort him, then I would cry and he would comfort me. We never really gave up hope. We spent hours with my husband's head on my belly trying to hear a heartbeat. All wind was taken as movement. It was not until she was born that we accepted that she was dead. I did not see her.

Some mothers, who have knowingly had to carry a dead baby inside them for 2 weeks or more, withdraw into themselves and try to suspend their feelings. A few have remained in this withdrawn state even after the birth of their next child. The causes for these different reactions are complex and can depend on a variety of reasons. It is always difficult at the time to know what is reaction to the death and what is a manifestation of previous difficulties.

Throughout this period of waiting for labor to begin, parents, especially mothers, can be helped by being given the opportunity to discuss their feelings and fears. Constantly talking about feelings and expressing emotions about what is happening can prevent a mother from withdrawing. Parents will need reassurance that the baby will not be decomposing rapidly inside the uterus. Some mothers fear that labor will be more difficult if "the baby will not be able to help itself." In fact, many of the dead babies are smaller than average, and labor is often easier. Because they are reluctant to "give birth to death" mothers may find it emotionally difficult to push their baby out.

> My labor was easy, but when I was told that I was able to push, my body did not feel the urge. The baby was in breech position so they fished his legs out and pulled. They seemed to think that the pain was bothering me but it was not. Again and again I was urged to push. I just could not push so I said, "Bloody hell, no that's not my job, I cannot." Then they seemed to understand and two nurses held a gas mask down over my face, I was shot full of local anesthetic and somehow they got the baby out.

In order to be able to verify their baby as a person, and to have someone tangible to mourn, parents need to see, and if possible to hold their dead baby. To some this idea is natural, to others is is abhorrent. Where the baby is known to be deformed or has been dead for some time parents may be scared to see their baby. It is worth remembering here that fears and fantasies are usually worse than reality and most parents are grateful later if they can talk about their fears and then be helped to see their baby. A photograph of the baby can be proof of its existence as later it can feel as though the whole event was a fantasy.

> As I did not have a baby and no one would speak of him I began to wonder if there really had been a baby. Had it really died of a knot in the cord or was it some hideous deformed monster? Who did it look like? If only someone had said, "He is perfectly formed—would you like to hold him?"

It is usually after the birth that the parents experience the deepest emotional pain. This is the time that they are most likely to cry. Death is the one time in adult life when tears are readily accepted and the person is still made to feel worthy. It is important that the newly bereaved parents are helped to feel that their grief is acceptable. Whereas most mothers do receive sympathy at this time, fathers' needs are often neglected. They can feel that they have to support their wives and try to continue normal life with little space allowed for their own grief. Parents need to be able to talk about their pain, to be encouraged to discuss their baby, and what its death means to them. This is the time when they will be asked to give consent for an autopsy. Most parents are eager to know what caused their baby's death and what implications this will hold for any future babies they plan. Some will not want the autopsy done. All will need to be able to discuss their feelings and secret fears, such as that the baby will not be made to "look nice" again after the autopsy. Parents have spoken of having strong guilt feelings after the autopsy was carried out despite having requested one.

At the time of delivery parents usually choose the least troublesome way of burying their babies. Later many wish they had had a funeral service of some sort, however simple. Funerals serve a twofold function. They mark a recognition not only of the respect due to the dead person, but also an acknowledgement of the chief mourners' loss and their need for comfort. Frequently parents find that there is a denial of their loss and therefore little comfort.

> Well it is not as though you knew him.
> Never mind dear, you are still young, you can always have another one next year to take its place. I felt as though I would scream if anyone else told me I could have another one. I wanted my baby! Whereas I was pleased to know that I could have another baby, I wanted *my* baby, not some mythical baby in the future.

Despite an apparent calm and even overt grieving over their baby's death, parents, especially mothers, may take as long as 3 months to accept that their baby is dead. Whereas this reaction is common and accepted when the dead person is a spouse whom the bereaved has known for a long time, it is not allowed for and hence not spoken about after a stillbirth. The denial of this and other normal grief reactions can lead to parents feeling that they have lost their sanity with their baby. They are usually only allowed a few weeks to grieve.

It is difficult to mourn a stillborn baby. Whether or not they want or expect to, parents find themselves grieving after the death of their baby. As they never knew their baby, they find themselves mourning someone who is intangible. Those who were able to hold their baby have a more real focus for their grief but even they are not always able to understand the intensity of their grief. Because of the intangible nature of their loss, feelings about previous unresolved losses can be reawakened and intensify their grief. This can make their reactions more bewildering and difficult to come to terms with.

Family and friends also can affect how parents react to a stillbirth. Parkes (1977) has suggested that bereaved who experience those around them as supportive tend to make a better adjustment to their loss than those who do not. Because of the difficulty of associating birth with death, and the fear of contamination, most parents find little support available to them. Bourne (1968) found that even their general practitioners had difficulty in dealing with parents. What parents tend to experience is a falling away of friends and relatives. This is probably because most people do not know what to say and tend to avoid the parents until they think they are "over it." Frequently, there is a denial of the importance of the event and in some cases a denial of the event itself.

> We were discussing labors. She was saying how much easier her second labor had been and how she thought everyone found this so. She turned to me and said "Of course you would not know anything about this." We had been working together for 6 years. My second child's birth/death had occurred 5 months previously. I was very hurt.

Where there are other pregnant women or mothers with small children in the parents' circle of friends, the reason given for withdrawing is to avoid upsetting the mother. However, Lewis (1979) has suggested that it is possible that they stay away because of a fear of being contaminated and having something happen to their children.

A stillbirth is frequently experienced as having failed in a basic human function, that of reproduction, and leads to feelings of inadequacy as a person. Usually this is felt most strongly by the mother. Often this feeling of inadequacy spills over into other areas of life.

> It was the first time I had ever failed to do something I really wanted to do. I felt that I would fail in everything else as well. I found myself unable to bake cakes, drive, or do many things I usually did.

Where genetic factors caused or influenced the baby's death, parents' feelings of inadequacy are increased: "I feel as though I have two ovaries full of damaged eggs." Going out and reestablishing old routines can be very painful. For many, it is their public acknowledgment that they have failed. Some women needed help going out for the first time. It can be very distressing to explain that you had a dead baby. If there is no one to help her, a mother may remain at home, ruminating over the event while the outside world grows more threatening. Most women find that when they do go their view of the population appears distorted. It is as though there are pregnant women or women with small babies everywhere.

> I thought I was going mad. Everywhere I went there were tiny babies. In the supermarket I was chased by a woman with a baby strapped in her front. I kept dodging behind counters, but everywhere I went, I saw her sailing down the passage-way towards me.

Many have strong feelings of envy about other pregnant women, some even wishing the same experience they had on these women. Because of the feeling that witchcraft and magic are around at the time of birth, and that these may account for their baby's death, these feelings of envy can be accompanied by a feeling of power and guilt usually leading to even greater feelings of inadequacy.

After the birth of their baby, many women, especially those who have other children, feel that their arms are empty, and that they need to cuddle something to fill them. Feelings about other newborn babies vary from that of longing and a desire to pick one up and keep it, to that of envy and of fear that they may harm the baby the way they harmed their own. Although these reactions are most common in mothers, some fathers also experience them. Parents may focus their normal grief reactions of anger and guilt on the hospital, its staff, the other parent, or on themselves.

> A father whose anencephalic baby was induced at 32 weeks blamed himself for what happened. He thought that anencephaly could occur only in females. As it is the man's sperm that determines the sex of the baby, he thought he was responsible for that particular baby being conceived and hence felt guilty and inadequate as a person. (After a few months he had a more rational attitude towards what had happened.)

Chance remarks, however lightheartedly they are made, can sharpen and deepen these feelings of guilt and anger.

> A mother, who was finding it difficult to manage her active toddler during her second pregnancy, decided to take him with her to spend a few weeks at her mother's. At the time she was 25 weeks pregnant. Shortly after arriving at her mother's home 400 miles away, she started bleeding and was admitted to hospital. A baby girl who only lived a few hours was born soon afterwards. Naturally she was very distressed. Later when she was back home she went for a check-up. Her doctor replied jokingly to the question "Why do you think it happened? Oh well, what else do you expect when you go traveling to the North like that." This was interpreted by the mother as all would have been well had she stayed at home and she redirected her anger and guilt onto herself.

As with all grief reactions, these should subside and be fitted into a perspective as the parents come to terms with their loss. Unfortunately, many parents strive to conceive another baby as quickly as possible. This may be following well-meant advice but often they do this in order to ease their feelings of inadequacy and pain. Many succeed and are given an expected date of delivery on or around the anniversary of their dead baby's birth. To mourn a stillbirth is partially to mourn the loss of a set of expectations about the way their lives will be changed by that baby. Lewis (1977) has suggested that it is difficult for parents to continue mourning their dead baby while they are expecting another baby that will have the same effect on their lives. If the next baby is conceived too soon, or if for some reason parents have been unable to grieve for their dead baby, mourning can be suspended during the subsequent pregnancy only to return after the birth of the next child.

> After the birth of my baby I mourned my failure to become the mother of two. I became pregnant as quickly as I could to ease the feeling of pain and failure. Once I was pregnant I felt better. Now that my next baby has been born I find myself mourning my dead little boy. I do not have the feeling of love for my little girl that I should have. No one seems to understand why I am not delighted and not forgetting about my dead baby now I have my new baby.

As already stated, mothers are allowed more time to grieve than are fathers. Fathers are expected to return to work and a normal routine very soon after the death of their baby. The normal demands of work, and the expectations that men will be strong and not show their emotions, gives fathers little time to express their grief. In addition, they are expected to provide the main support for their wives. This disparity of expectations and behavior can lead to problems in the marriage after the initial period of mutual support. Where the wife was previously the stronger partner the burden of carrying her can be too much for the father: "You are no longer fun the way you were when we got married." He may withdraw and even leave the marriage. In the latter case, the mother will find her grief intensified without being able to sort out what belongs to the baby and what to the break-up of the marriage. She will also be very bitter. Fortunately, this happens rarely. Usually impatience at the wife's continuing grief and anger at the husband's apparent lack of caring will be expressed and the couple will bicker more. Changes may also occur in the couple's pattern of sexual relations. These can vary from demanding sexual intercourse regularly as soon after the birth as is possible in order to gain reassurance of still being desirable, and hence not totally inadequate as a woman, to not being able to participate "in the act that resulted in a baby's death." Once the next pregnancy has been started, the bickering appears to cease. Because they have both failed in having a baby, couples who might previously have been moving towards a separation, tend to stay together until they have safely had their next child. In marriages where one partner has children from a previous union, extra stress can be placed on the marriage.

"You could have his child, why not mine?"

The most difficult death to mourn is that of a stillborn twin when the other baby is alive and well. Everyone rejoices at the birth of the live baby. The mother frequently does not even have the understanding and support of her husband in her grief over their loss. She feels isolated in her own family. Often the mother visualizes the dead child alongside the surviving twin for many years. She may blame the surviving twin for the death of the other one. Professional counseling should always be offered to these parents. The points to be worked through are the same as in other stillbirths. The family has to be helped to understand the mother's need for acknowledgement of the importance to her of the existence of the other twin, to enable her to concentrate on the living.

If parents already have a child, it is expected that they will find comfort in it. "Never mind, you have already got one at home. Just think of those who cannot have any all." Most parents do find it comforting to care for their other children but many become overprotective of their children and make them their excuse for living. However, some are resentful when their children make demands on them and intrude into their thoughts and feelings about the dead baby. Later they may become overprotective. A common reaction after a stillbirth is that of regression: of wanting to be cuddled and cared for. It is difficult to regress when there is a child to care for, especially one who is frightened and bewildered and hence very demanding. This is a time when a small child needs extra care and attention as its parents no longer appear to be able to take charge of its world. A small child will not be able to sort out whether any of its thoughts affected what happened to the baby. Inadequate explanations, rejection, or a denial that anything important has happened can lead to fears and behavioral problems later.

> At the time our 3-year-old said very little. He did not seem to want to know or care very much, as long as I was okay. I had the definite feeling that he had not wanted the rotten baby anyway and was glad to be let off the hook. We foolishly assumed he was too young to care very much and I was too sad and grief-stricken to meet his needs fully. Great problems and jealously experienced with him for almost 2 years after the birth of our next child the following year made us wonder if he had felt confused, possibly guilty, that his lack of enthusiasm had killed the baby. Certainly the problems eased after we had gently probed the subject, let him talk and reassured him. He still says very little, though if we meet a handicapped child, he often asks "Was Elisabeth like that?"

An interesting phenomenon in that is many cases the children do not show their reactions until some time after the baby's death. It is as though they are waiting for their parents to regain their emotional strength. Many become extremely anxious during the pregnancy even when it was thought that they were too young to know what was happening at the time.

The difficulty parents have in mourning their dead baby once the next baby has been conceived has already been mentioned. Most find the next pregnancy an extremely anxious time, with the mother showing the most overt anxiety. However, because it is expected that she will be happy after having conceived again, little emotional support is offered although she is usually assured of good medical attention. Some parents manage by projecting their anxiety onto those around them while they sail unconcernedly through the pregnancy. Most are not as fortunate. It is difficult for anxious parents to prepare emotionally or practically for a live baby. This is because they are expecting to give birth to death again, and even if the baby lives they may have difficulty in accepting that it will remain alive. This difficulty can be exacerbated if the baby has problems at birth or has to be treated in a special care baby unit.

> I felt unable to push my baby out. I knew that she would not cry when she was born—that she would be dead. The baby was fine.

> I insisted on having an epidural for the cesarean section because I "knew" my baby would be born dead and I was determined to cuddle this one. When he was safely delivered I burst into tears of relief. He was taken up to the special care unit to go into an incubator as he was only a 35-week baby. In the recovery room I settled down to wait for him to die. I was not aware of it at the time, and I think that I only accepted that he was going to live when he was 6 or 7 months old. I breastfed him determinedly and did all the right things that are supposed to lead to forming a strong bond with a baby, but it was not until someone remarked that he had a sense of humor when he was about 6 months old that I accepted that he was a person here to stay.

Some parents, especially when the time gap between the birth of two babies is very short, expect the new baby to be both babies, in one. Others expect the new baby to catch up to what the dead baby would have been doing had it lived.

> My baby is refusing the breast at the midday feed. She is only 4 months old. I am extremely upset. She does not seem to realize that she is feeding for both of them. The other one would not have refused to nurse so early.

There is an expectation that the birth of the next baby will make up for the stillbirth. From what has already been said, it is clear that frequently this does not happen. In many cases, the next baby and time do ease the pain and the nightmare quality of the event. The stillbirth fades into a painful experience in the past, although anniversaries can revive feelings. However, for some parents the stillbirth can remain the most important event of their life with the pain, inadequacies and anxiety it unleashed continuing to influence their lives.

Until recently there was little understanding of the effects of a stillbirth and hence little support available to bereaved parents. Interest in bereavement and its effects has grown in the last decade. This has led to more awareness of the needs of parents who have suffered a stillbirth. Some hospitals have bereavement clinics where parents can go for counseling. Such clinics are few. In other areas, local women have banded together to offer a service to the newly bereaved such as A.M.E.N.D. in St Louis, Missouri. In Great Britain, the national stillbirth association has been formed.[1] It aims to improve knowledge available on the causes and effects of stillbirths and other perinatal deaths. It also operates a national supportive network for parents who have suffered a perinatal death. The association is in the process of setting up local groups that will develop liaisons with maternity units and be able to offer support to all newly bereaved parents. Each group has advisors in the psychiatric and obstetric fields to whom they can turn for advise. Of the first 100 women referred to the association in 1979, not one refused the support offered although some husbands felt that they did not require help. The National Stillbirth Study Group (1979) has drawn up a leaflet which the Health Education Council has published and distributed to all obstetric units in Great Britain. This should improve the information available to parents at the time of their bereavement and make it a less isolating and bewildering experience.

[1]The Stillbirth and Perinatal Death Association is located at 15a Christchurch Hill, London, NW3, IJY, England.

The Stillbirth and Perinatal Death Association (1979) has drawn up guidelines to help parents who wish to befriend and offer support to the newly bereaved. It is hoped that through offering support, and where necessary professional help, parents will be better able to come to terms with their loss and avoid some of the problems mentioned above.

REFERENCES

Bourne, S. The psychological effects of stillbirths on women and their doctors. *Journal of the Royal College of General Practioners,* 1968, *16,* 103–112.

Lewis, E. The inhibition of mourning by pregnancy. Scientific Notice Board, Institute of Psychoanalysis, December 1977, 24–26.

Lewis, H. Nothing was said sympathy wise, they looked after me, but never comforted me. *Social Work Today,* 1979, *10,* 12–13.

National Stillbirth Study Group. Stillbirth and neonatal death. London: Health Education Council, 1979.

Parkes, C. M. Evaluation of family care in terminal illness. In E. Prichard & J. Collard (Eds.). *Social work with the dying patient in the family.* New York: Columbia University Press, 1977.

Stillbirth Association. Notes on initial visit by a befriending parent. London: Stillbirth Association, 1979.

BIBLIOGRAPHY

Anthony, S. *The discovery of death in childhood and after.* London: Penguin, 1973.

Beard, R. Help for parents after a stillbirth. *British Medical Journal,* 1978, *1,* 172–173.

Bruce, S. J. Reactions of nurses and mothers to stillbirths. *Nursing Outlook,* 1962, *10,* 88–91.

Cain, A. C., & Cain, B. S. On replacing a child. *Journal of American Academic Child Psychiatry,* 1964, *3,* 43–48.

Cain, A. C., Erickson, M. E., Fast, I., Vaughan, R. Children's disturbed reactions to their miscarriage. *Psychosomatic Medicine,* 1964, *26,* 58–66.

Cain A. C., Fast, I., Erickson, M. E. Children's disturbed reaction to the death of a sibling. *American Journal of Orthopsychiatry, 34,* 741–752.

Giles, F. Reaction of women to perinatal death. *Australian and New Zealand Journal of Obstretrics and Gynecology,* 1970, *10,* 207–210.

Jolly, H. Family reactions to stillbirth. *Proceedings of the Royal Society of Medicine,* 1976, *69,* 835–837.

Kennell, J. A. *Maternal infant bonding.* St. Louis: Mosby, 1976.

Kitzinger, S. Counselling after a stillbirth. *Marriage Guidance,* 1976, 39–45.

Lewis, E. The management of stillbirth: Coping with an unreality. *Lancet,* 1975, *ii,* 619–620.

Lewis, H. Difficulties in mourning and stillbirth. *New Society* (in press, 1980).

Morris, D. Parental reactions to perinatal death. *Proceedings of the Royal Society of Medicine,* 1976, *69,* 837–838.

Parkes, C. M. Health after bereavement. *Psychiatric Medicine,* 1972, *34,* 449–461.

Seitz, P. M. Perinatal death: the grieving mother. *American Journal of Nursing,* 1974, *74,* 2028–2033.

Wyss, M. Patterns of grief in a mother experiencing newborn death. *Leaflet for A.M.E.N.D.* St Louis, 1978.

chapter 20

THE NATURE AND FUNCTION OF EARLY MOTHER-INFANT INTERACTION

Gail Wasserman

So far as the child's mind is concerned, the fond delusion which mothers commonly cherish, that children perceive and recognize as soon as born, or soon after birth, must be disregarded. It is probably not before the third or fourth month of infancy that the human being perceives. By this we mean that while rays of light may fall upon the child's eyes, and waves of sound may strike its ears, and sensations of cold or warmth or roughness or smoothness be excited in its skin, and while sound may be heard as confused noise, yet the child has no idea as to the meaning, source, or character of these sensations.

(Davis & Keating, 1892)

The rule that parents should not play with the young baby may seem hard, but it is without doubt a safe one. A young, delicate, or nervous baby especially needs rest and quiet, and however robust the child much of the play that is indulged in is more or less harmful. . . . The mother should not kiss the baby directly on the mouth. . . . as infections of various kinds are spread in this way. She needs also to be cautioned about rocking the baby.

(West, 1914)

Certainly our view of both the very young infant and of the optimal setting for his development has changed immeasurably since these early descriptions. Over the last several years, developmental psychologists have been observing and documenting evidence for earlier and earlier infant capacities. Some fruitful lines of research have investigated the capacities available to the infant, even before birth. Evidence concerning both prenatal behavior and the behavior of premature infants at less than 40 weeks postconception suggests that the infant is exposed to and responsive to human and nonhuman stimulation far earlier than was previously imagined (MacFarlane, 1977; Miranda, 1970; Robinson, 1966; Sontag and Wallace, 1935; Spelt, 1938, 1948).

The neonatal period is usually, however, the earliest time when we can begin to examine behavior. From an ethological perspective, the period of early infancy is ideal for the examination of species-specific behavior before major learning has taken place.

From the earliest period, the infant shows evidence of a network of capacity and responsiveness to the behavior and stimulus characteristics of those around him. This network firmly roots him in his species, and aids in the development of social ties between him and his caregivers. Not only is the infant primed to attend to his social world, but members of that social world are clearly tuned in to his presence and special needs as well. These behavioral systems, which are characteristic of the species at large, are likely biological in nature. They aid in the survival of the species, since it is clearly necessary for the helpless human infant to have others around for him to thrive and survive. Through natural selection, these biobehavioral systems have become part of the genetic makeup of our species. Bardwick (1974) suggests that what is inherited is not the behavior itself, but rather, the capacity to develop a behavioral system: "the nature and the form of the developed behavioral system will be a joint function of the inherent capacity to develop and the particular environment in which development takes place." This chapter will first discuss the nature of this early interactional system, and will then go on to discuss some current research on the infant's early language environment as an example of the way in which such interactions operate.

EARLY INFANT SOCIAL RESPONSIVENESS

Hearing

Newborn infants show discriminative alerting towards a female voice; when placed between a male and a female speaker, the newborn tends to orient his head in the direction of the female (Brazelton, personal communication, 1976). Similar results have been reported for responses to tones in the range of the female voice (Hutt, 1973; Kearsley, 1973). Both of these tendencies are present in the first days after birth, when we may assume that the infant has not yet learned to associate the female voice with any "reward" or comfort. While these investigations do not rule out prenatal exposure, we would first need to analyze the prenatal environment to determine whether the majority of voices to which the infant is exposed in utero are female. Further, even if the infant is exposed to more high-pitched voices, the development of such early discriminative and responsive capacities prior to birth is an awesome finding in itself.

Infants in a newborn nursery cry less when exposed to a metronome running at 72 beats per minute (Salk, 1973). This rate corresponds to human adult heart rate, and Salk contends that infants are imprinted upon this rhythm as a result of extended exposure to the mother's heart beat prior to birth, and that they find it comforting even after separation from the prenatal environment.

By 2 weeks after birth, infants show more smiling in response to a high-pitched voice than to other stimuli (Wolff,

1963). This occurs whether the speaker is a female or a male employing the falsetto range. Actual discriminatory smiling to the mother's voice, as opposed to other female voices, comes rather later, and postnatal experience can be presumed to play an important role here. The early predisposition to respond to human voices, as opposed to other sounds, can then be redefined and strengthened as the infant continues to experience interactions with those around him.

Vision

As early as 9 minutes after birth, infants will track a moving 2-dimensional representation of a face by moving their heads and eyes. Such head and eye turning is significantly more likely to appear with face-like stimuli than with scrambled faces or with blank circles (Goren, Sarty, Wu, 1975). Similarly, a representation of the human face elicits more visual fixation (and inferentially, greater "preference") than a colored disk, a bull's eye, newsprint, a red square, or a lighted orange globe (Fantz, 1963, 1965, 1967). While this is often considered as evidence for an innate preference or innate recognition of facelike qualities, others have suggested that the early responsivity of the infant to the dimensions of facelike stimuli can be explained on the basis of reactions to or preferences for a given amount of contrast, contour, movement, or complexity (Bond, 1972; Caron et al., 1973; Haaf & Bell, 1967; Hershenson, Kessen, Munsinger, 1967).

Whatever the dimensions of this early responsivity, by the 7th day of life infants are sufficiently capable of discriminating the familiar so that when their mothers feed them silently while wearing a surgical mask, they take less milk and show subsequent disruption in rapid eye movement–(REM)–and non-REM–sleep (Cassell & Sander, 1975). By 2 weeks, an infant can discriminate his mother's face from either a three-dimensional model of a face or a three-dimensional nonface stimulus (Carpenter, 1974) and by 1 month of age, he can discriminate his mother's face from that of a female stranger (Maurer & Salapa-tek, 1976). Interestingly enough, such discrimination is mani-fested by *less* looking at the mother than at other stimuli, and probably reflects some early habituation to the familiar features of the mother's face.

Certainly, maintaining eye contact with her infant is very important for a mother (Robson, 1967) and the infant very likely associates his view of the face with some positive feelings on his own part as well as with some positive response to emotional feedback from the mother. This association may arise because the infant views the face either during the feeding situation or in the context of play (Watson, 1972). By 4 weeks of age, infants demonstrate the positive, attractive value of faces by smiling; at this age there is more smiling to human faces than to other stimuli (Spitz & Wolf, 1946). Nevertheless, as was the case with his auditory responsiveness, evidence exists from these earliest days that human faces are of great interest to the infant. This early "set" toward such visual stimuli is elaborated, amplified, and given social meaning by the events occuring over the first weeks and months of the infant's life.

Smell and Taste

Less evidence is available for smell or taste discriminations which have interactional implications than is the case for hear-ing or vision. One provocative finding is that by 5 days of life an infant can tell the difference between a gauze pad which has been worn next to the breast by his nursing mother and that worn by another mother. The infant shows that he can discrimi-nate between these two very similar odors by orienting in the direction of his mother's pad (MacFarlane, 1975).

Movement

Newborn infants respond with subtle movement patterns to the rhythms and stresses of human speech (Condon &

Sander, 1974). This synchrony between adult speech and infant movement can be detected by slow motion analysis of filmed interactions and occurs also with dialogues between two adults. Newborn infants do not respond with such synchronized movement to nonhuman patterned sounds.

In summary, the young infant shows in many ways that he comes into this world equipped to respond to members of his own species. His behavior, while not consciously or even voluntarily social in the first days of life, is nonetheless oriented toward other human beings. Over the next several weeks, months, and years such initial tendencies are expanded, differentiated, and given meaning by the interaction in which this growing person engages.

EARLY SOCIAL RESPONSIVENESS TO INFANTS

If there is evidence that the infant comes equipped to orient to his species, and perhaps especially to the female members of his species, there is also the suggestion that mothers, and perhaps fathers as well, are especially responsive to the cues given out by the infant in the earliest days after birth. Klaus and Kennell (1976) have elaborated several principles central to what they have termed "bonding," in referring to the mother's (and father's) role in the relationship with the infant. Most basically, these authors suggest that the first few hours after birth constitute a "sensitive period" for the development of the mother–infant relationship. They suggest that exposure to the infant at this time is necessary for later optimal development of the bond. Further, anxieties about early temporary difficulties in bonding may become lasting concerns that adversely affect development.

The investigations offered as support for an early "sensitive period" have sufficient methodological difficulties to cause us to withhold judgment at this time. The development of a significant social bond between the infant and his caregivers is of such great importance to the survival of our species that its presence must surely be overdetermined and biologically buffered. The first few hours after birth constitute only one of many opportunities for the emergence of such a bond, as indicated above. However, this is not to say that the kinds of disruptions that occur after the birth of a potentially or actually damaged infant do not have importance for the subsequent emergence of responsive fine-tuning in the mother–infant system. When the separation is long, and especially when it is coupled with the reality of illness and anxiety about the infant's future development, there may very well be disturbances in mother–infant interaction (Stern & Wasserman, 1979).

While we may show some skepticism about the necessity of an early critical period in setting down a vital mother–infant relationship, there is much evidence that suggests a high degree of fine-tuning from the earliest days in that relationship. Mother and infant operate within a very sensitive feedback system; the behavior of each of them is maintained by instant control of responses and cues coming from the other. Without this, we would not have the synchrony and reciprocity suggested by Brazelton et al. (1974), Condon and Sander (1974), and Stern (1977). As was the case with infant behavior, most research on maternal behavior with very young infants has centered around visual and auditory behaviors.

Visual Stimulation

As indicated above, mothers find eye contact with their infants rewarding from the first few days of the infant's life (Klaus et al., 1970; Robson, 1967). In fact, the mother looks at her infant almost all the time when they are interacting (Stern, 1974), a pattern which differs from that occurring in other dyadic situations. The tendency of mothers to maintain an "en face" position during an interaction thus coincides with the established early preferences for human faces as opposed to other visual stimuli: the infant "prefers" to look at faces.

Aside from this greater likelihood of presenting a facial stimulus to the infant, mothers are also more likely to offer dynamic visual stimulation which seems unique to interactions with infants. Thus, Stern et al. (1977) and Stern & Gibbon (1979) report that the kinesthetic aspects of the caregiver's facial and bodily display show a high level of exaggeration, repetitiveness, and rhythmicity not found in other interactions. The role of these factors will be elaborated in greater detail below.

One consistent human response to interesting visual information is that of pupil dilation. Not only do people show preferences for photographs of infants as opposed to adults[1] (Cann, 1969), they also show greater pupillary responses to the more "babyish" photographs (Hess, 1967). This quality of "babyishness," then, has appeal to those around the infant and most likely is of high survival value, insuring that others will find the infant of interest and worthy of caregiving (Hess, 1969).

Those who interact with the infant thus behave in ways that appear to be geared to his capacities and preferences. The patterning of such behavior directed toward infants appears to be sufficiently unique as to warrant the summary label of "parenting behavior." Parallels are easily discovered between these unique "infant-elicited" (Stern, 1977) behaviors in the visual system and functionally similar behaviors in the auditory system.

Auditory Stimulation

Salk (1973) has commented on the tendency of mothers, regardless of handedness, to hold the infant in the left arm, thus keeping him exposed to the maternal heartbeat, the sound of which presumably acts to soothe the infant. Most observations of maternal accommodations to the infant's particular auditory

[1]Actually, this is consistently the case only for women. Preferences of men depend upon experiences with parenting.

preferences and responsiveness, however, have been concerned with mothers' language. Investigations of the way in which mothers talk to their infants over the first few months of life provide us with a model which may allow us to understand better the function and developmental change in all such infant-elicited behavioral systems. The results of some of our current research on maternal language over the first 6 months of life will be considered next.

THE INFANT'S LANGUAGE ENVIRONMENT

One common observation concerning the way parents talk to their young infants (and the way those infants respond) is that the *way* something is said is of greater importance than exactly *what* is said. It has been suggested (Stern & Wasserman, in preparation) that the prosodic features (the "music" of what the mother says) play a larger role early in the infant's life than does the actual content of what she says (the "lyrics") in transmitting affective signals, in marking the boundaries within the flow of speech, and in focusing and regulating an interaction. In preparing to investigate these issues, it was presumed that systematic study of the prosodic features (intonation contour, timing, repetition, and rhythm) of maternal speech directed to infants over their earliest months might reveal a sequence of changes that would provide us with information about both the infant's perceptual capacities, as well as about the ways in which mother–infant interchanges are determined.

Study 1

Samples of the speech of six mothers of healthy infants were collected, while mothers and infants were engaged in a play session. In order to control for the effects of experience, all infants were firstborn,[2] and all mothers were native speakers of American English. Mother–infant pairs were seen in the first days after birth, and again at 2, 4, and 6 months as part of a continuing longitudinal study of maternal styles and infant social development. Several aspects of maternal language were then coded. While all features of maternal language to infants differed from the language samples of the same mothers' speech directed toward adults, it is the developmental aspects of mothers' language to infants that will be discussed here.

TIMING.   It has been suggested (e.g., Snow, 1977) that mothers speak more slowly when addressing infants. In order to examine this issue, audiotape recordings were played through a polygraph and pen deflections corresponding to the vocalizations themselves were measured, generating information on the duration of maternal vocalizations (corresponding to continuous utterances), pauses, and the vocalization-plus-pause-interval (an utterance plus its subsequent pause). Over the ages studied, the vocalization-plus-pause-interval decreases, and this can be accounted for by age related changes in pause length (see Fig.20.1a). In other words, *mothers' speech is most slow with newborns and it gets progressively faster as the infant gets older.*

RHYTHM.   Mothers' speech to young infants has been found to be especially rhythmic (e.g., Blount & Padgug, 1977). In investigating changes in that rhythmicity over the first 6 months of life, the measure used was the coefficient of variation (the $sd/\bar{x}$) of the vocalization-plus-pause-interval. This assesses the regularity of the beat of mothers' language. The smaller the coefficient of variation, the tighter the rhythm. *The rhythm of*

---

[2]We have also established the lack of any differences in either the developmental emergence or the patterning of the behaviors, to be described below, as a function of parity: mothers behave in virtually identical fashion regardless of whether the infants with whom they are interacting is their first- or second-born.

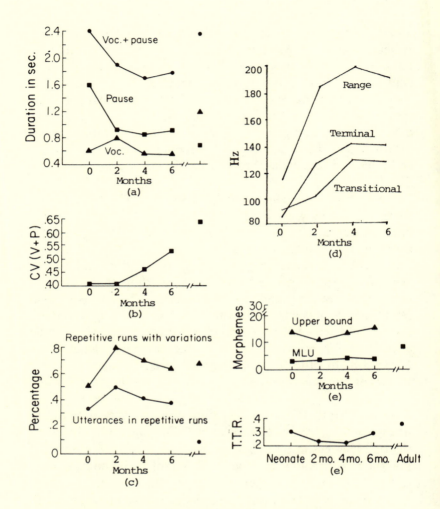

Fig. 20-1. Changes over infant age in maternal language: (a) timing, (b) rhythm, (c) repetition, (d) intonation, and (e) complexity.

mothers' speech, as indicated in Figure 20.1b, is tightest with newborns and 2-month-olds, and becomes increasingly variable as the infant gets older.

REPETITION. Previous research (e.g., Snow, 1972) has found repetitiveness to be a salient characteristic of maternal language. For this investigation, two measures of repetition were examined: The percentage of utterances in repetitive runs (strings of repetitive vocalizations) and the percentage of repetitive runs with variations (those which are slightly different from one vocalization to the next). As Figure 20–1c shows, *mothers are most repetitive with infants when they are 2 months old.*

INTONATION. Anecdotal evidence suggests that maternal speech to infants is characterized by exaggerated pitch contouring. The tapes were, therefore, processed through a narrow band filter sound spectrograph which isolated the continuously changing fundamental frequency of the maternal vocalizations. This is the same sort of equipment used to produce a visual record of birdsong. Whether we examine the last unidirectional pitch change in each utterance ("terminal change"), the degree of pitch change from one maternal utterance to the next ("transitional change"), or the difference between the highest and lowest points in each utterance ("range"), *there is evidence of increasing use of pitch contouring as the infant grows older* (Fig. 20-1d).

COMPLEXITY. While the nonprosodic elements of language directed to infants are likely to be very different from language directed to adults, no developmental changes are apparent in the way mothers use this aspect of speech. Over the ages studied, Mean Length of Utterance (average number of morphenes per utterance), Upper Bound (number of morphenes in longest utterance), and Type-Token Ratio (variability in vocabulary) revealed no differences (Fig.20-1e).

The Function of Age-Related Changes in Maternal Language

The findings indicate that there are age-related changes in prosodic but not in the syntactic features of maternal speech to infants during the first 6 months of life. During this period, the prosodic features do not change at the same time; rather, different elements appear to be more or less emphasized at different ages. The data point to an age-related sequence, shown schematically in Figure 20-2, which can be summarized briefly as follows: *During the neonatal period the timing and rhythm of the maternal language behavior are most emphasized (emphasized in the sense of diverging from the adult norm); by 2 months of age the extent of maternal repetitions and the continued regularity of rhythm characterize the period; between 4 and 6 months, accentuated intonation contours are characteristic; and at some*

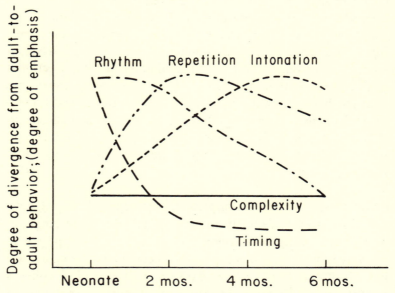

Fig. 20-2. Schematic representation of the sequence of developmental phases in the emphasis of various prosodic features of the infant's language environment.

point after 6 months, when the infant begins to understand and learn language, we expect that syntactic changes will occupy the foreground.

In a social interaction, the mother's behavior is largely under the instant-by-instant feedback control from the infant and vice versa. Maternal behavior, therefore, can be expected to match aspects of the infant's perceptual and response capabilities. Investigating age-related changes in maternal behavior, then, allows us to examine the timetable for the unfolding of infant abilities. We would suggest that these changes can be conceptualized as a sequence of developmental phases in the infant's perception of and response to the prosodic features of human speech.

During the neonatal period, compared to all other ages, the elongation of pauses is relatively greater, resulting in a longer beat interval and a slower tempo. We speculate that the maternal language behavior is geared to the infant's immature stimulus (and information) and processing abilities, in the sense that long pauses permit more processing time before the next "chunk" arrives.

By 2 months, the infant's processing speed and capabilities have progressed so that he is able to handle the temporal auditory stimulus pattern of burst-pause that will obtain through the later developmental stages studied. Even though the information he extracts from each stimulus may expand constantly, the relative and absolute timing of stimulus presentations will change little. A second major "event" during the 2-month period is that the amount of maternal repetitions reaches its peak. From our data and the reports of Blount and Padgug (1977); Dunn, Wooding, & Hermann (1977); and Snow (1972), it appears that repetitions reach their peak around 2 months and then follow a gradual decline over the next few years. A third feature characteristic of the 2-month period is the regularity of the rhythm of maternal utterances. Only after 2 months does this strictness of beat begin to loosen and approach adult levels. The two features of repetition and regularity of beat that mark this 2-month phase may act together to provide the infant with a particular format or presentation of human speech signals of importance to infant learning. The high degree of repetition permits the infant to exercise his tendency to create and to test expectancies about the qualities of the stimulus he can now anticipate hearing. The progressive introduction of variations in repetitive runs permits him to evaluate discrepancies from the expected. At the same time, the tight rhythm permits him to both create and test temporal expectancies (of when the next stimulus might be expected to occur).

Between the 4th and 6th month of life, the exaggeration in intonation contour peaks, while the emphasis on timing, rhythm, and repetitions have begun to subside. A later developmental data point would be required to determine subsequent changes in intonation contouring. The data thus far suggest that the mother may be responding to an advance in the infant's developmental readiness to discriminate and respond to the intonational features of the speech signal. Certainly the experimental evidence of Chang & Trehub (1977), Kuhl (1976), and Morse (1972) showing infant discrimination of pitch changes within the first 6 months is compatible with this shift in emphasis.

It is widely thought that a significant part of the vocal expression of affect is carried in the degree and speed of changes in fundamental voice frequency (e.g., Sherrer, 1974). Because of his increased ability to discriminate pitch contours during this 4–6-month phase, the infant may be learning to discriminate different emotions as they are expressed vocally. It has been suggested that by 6 months infants are capable of discriminating various emotional facial displays (Charlesworth & Kreutzer, 1973). Perhaps the early discrimination of emotions, as expressed both vocally and visually, begins to take place at this time, such that the bimodal integration of affect recognition is assured.

Finally, at some point beyond the 6th month of life the semantic and syntactic features of the infant's language environment begin to change radically as language production becomes manifest. By this time, however, it is probable that the infant has already learned much about the nature of speech timing, rhythm, sounds, and intonational contours.

The Regulation of Attention, Arousal, and Affect

The major goals of the mother during a social interaction with her infant are first to attract and hold his attention and, second, to elicit signals, such as smiles, coos, and the like, which indicate that the infant is in a state of moderate arousal and positive affect. In order to accomplish this as the infant matures, she must adapt the quality and quantity of her social behavior to stay in step with her infant. The kind of stimulation that is effective in getting and holding the attention of a newborn and in keeping his level of excitement well modulated will be too simple, too slow, and too mild for maintaining a lively interaction with an older infant. On the other hand, the relatively more complicated, faster, and more intense stimulation required to maintain a smoothly regulated interaction with a 6-month-old would prove overstimulating to a much younger infant. The mother is required, then, if she wishes to maintain an interactive match with her infant, to introduce age-related changes in all her behaviors, including language behavior.

In order to maintain infant attention, arousal, and affect at levels appropriate to positive social interchange, the mother makes use of a theme-and-variations format of stimulus presentation (Stern et al., 1977). She presents a stimulus (some piece of behavior) to the infant, evaluates its immediate effect on the interaction, and uses this information in producing her next stimulus. As long as a stimulus is effective (provided the mother does not tire of the game), it will be repeated. If the infant's level of attention or arousal threatens to wane, the mother must respond with some slight variation, or a whole new pattern of theme-and-variations.

The age-related changes in the prosodic features of mothers' language, therefore, seem well-suited for the regulation of a social interaction. First, the quality of stimulation offered varies over the first 6 months in the direction of increased stimulation: stimulus density (shorter pauses), speed (faster tempo), intensity (accentuation of intonation contours), variability of temporal and auditory patterning (relaxation of the strictness of beat and repetitions with variations). Second, the vocalization and pause pattern, the regular (although somewhat variable) intervals between stimuli, and the degree of repetition, provide the mother with the necessary elements to fashion a theme-and-variations format for stimulus presentation.

Teaching the Conversational Mode

As Snow (1977) has suggested, a vocal interchange between a mother and an infant is conversational in nature. Not only is much of the mother's behavior directed towards eliciting responses from the infant, but mothers interpret burps, yawns, sneezes, and smiles as communicative actions on the part of the baby. If the infant does not respond, the mother may even take his turn (Stern et al., 1975; Stern, 1977). If the infant is to become a true turntaking conversational partner, he must know when the turn has been passed to him. He must learn to chunk the input from the mother's speech so that he can differentiate between pauses occurring in between words within a continuous utterance (non-turn-switching pauses) and those occurring between the utterances themselves (turn-switching pauses). The infant's "turn" to respond comes in the spaces between maternal vocalizations. The mother helps the infant to accomplish this task by making turntaking invitational pauses very long relative to those occurring within a burst of speech, during the first 2 months of life. The elongated pauses provide a longer period both for the slower processing speed of the young infant and also allow the infant to slip in a response in the time allotted for his turn.

In addition, the presence of terminal pitch changes provides the infant with cues marking the ends of utterances in a way that is exaggerated in comparison to the adult-to-adult mode. Transitional pitch changes (across potential turn-taking pauses) may help the infant distinguish that a new utterance has begun and is a different event, i.e., not a continuation, even after a pause, of the preceding utterance. In summary, the infant receives much repeated experience in which the onset and offset of potential turn-switching pauses are highly marked. It is not suggested here that mothers perform any of these prosodic features in order to enhance the infant's developing ability to participate in the conversational mode, but only that such an enhancement is the likely outcome of her behavior.

Study 2

The underlying assumption of all mother–infant interaction research, and certainly the central thrust of the previous argument, is that we anticipate a great deal of alignment between maternal and infant behavior. It can be presumed that the presence of a considerable level of deviancy in the infant would result in qualitative and quantitative differences in maternal interactive styles.

Accordingly, in order to examine the differential role of infant input into the mother–infant system, the interactions of infants who are at risk for central nervous system damage and their mothers were observed. Six subjects, all of whom were "graduates" of New York Hospital's Neonatal Intensive Care Unit, were followed. All infants were of low birth weight (less than 2000 grams), premature (less than 32 weeks gestation), and had spent time on a respirator. Their at-risk status was confirmed by developmental evaluations at 6 months: even when corrections were made for prematurity, the mean Bayley score in this group was 76, as opposed to 118 for the control population.

Once again, tape recordings of mother and infant at play were collected at 0, 2, 4, and 6 months (age-corrected). Because these at-risk infants were a combined group of first- and later-borns, they were compared to a control group of mixed parity. In comparing the control and at-risk samples, two patterns were found. First, rhythm and timing of maternal vocalizations in mothers of at-risk infants grow more and more similar to those of control mothers as the infants grow older (Fig.20-3).

RHYTHM.   The rhythm of speech in mothers of at-risk infants is most different from that of control mothers at the newborn stage. The rhythm is looser with the at-risk group (Fig.20-3a). The convergence over age seems to indicate that this language feature is a basic baby-elicited behavior that may be independent of the risk status of the infant.

TIMING.   The timing of mothers' speech with at-risk infants is especially different when those infants are 2 months old (Fig.20-3b). The pattern which appears is the reverse of what would be expected in this case, since these mothers are actually talking *faster* to their infants than are mothers of control infants, although the differences between groups diminish with age. Perhaps the mother uses a pattern of shorter pauses because she does not know when to stop and start her utterances because the usual cues of expression and gaze pattern may be less evident with an infant who is considered "at-risk" (Cicchetti & Sroufe, 1978; Emde, Katz, & Thorpe, 1978). The mother may also be talking faster because she is "filling time" in interacting with an unresponsive baby.

A second pattern appears with repetition and intonation. In both these features, mothers of at-risk infants diverge increasingly from the control norms with increasing infant age.

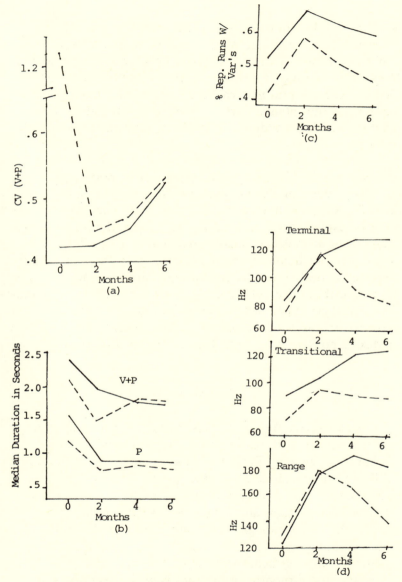

Fig. 20-3. Comparisons between mothers of at-risk and control infants in (a) rhythm, (b) timing, (c) repetition, and (d) intonation.

343

REPETITION.   As can be seen in Fig.20-3c, the degree of repetitiveness in the language of the mother of the at-risk infant differs from that of the control mother after the infant age of 2 months. The use of repetitions with variations probably reflects a more playful maternal style and is likely geared to an ability, on the infant's part, to process cognitively dissonant stimuli. Neither condition is likely to prevail in the at-risk infant.

INTONATION.   While the contouring curves for both samples are virtually identical during the newborn and 2-month period (Fig.20-3d), they diverge sharply after that. These results can best be explained by considering once again the link between contouring and affect expression and maintenance. The increasing lack of such contouring may reflect both the mother's depression in dealing with an increasingly obviously deviant child as well as the absence of the kind of cues coming from the infant and contingent upon her own behavior that allow her to remain positive and aroused. Intonation, then, seems to be a sensitive index of positive involvement at a high level of arousal.

SUMMARY

In summary then, the investigation of maternal language reveals several features important for the study of maternal behavior in general. First, the language directed to the infant differs from that directed to other adults, in that the former is less complex, more repetitious, more rhythmic, and consists of shorter vocalizations and longer pauses. On a qualitative level, it sounds unique enough to warrant consideration as a variety of "parenting behavior." Second, the emergence of features of maternal language behavior shows a developmental progression over the first 6 months of life that is well-integrated with the appearance, in the infant, of certain response capacities and preferences. Additionlly, both in degree and in pattern of emer-

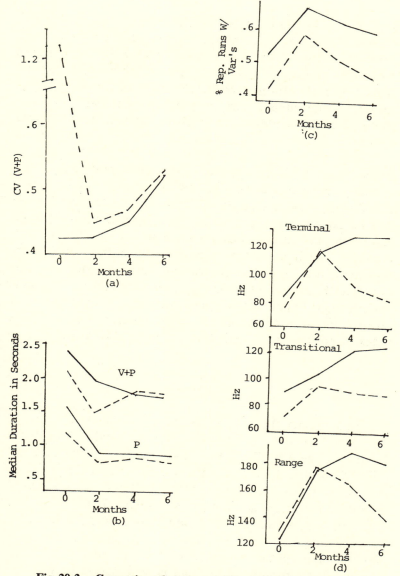

Fig. 20-3. Comparisons between mothers of at-risk and control infants in (a) rhythm, (b) timing, (c) repetition, and (d) intonation.

REPETITION. As can be seen in Fig.20-3c, the degree of repetitiveness in the language of the mother of the at-risk infant differs from that of the control mother after the infant age of 2 months. The use of repetitions with variations probably reflects a more playful maternal style and is likely geared to an ability, on the infant's part, to process cognitively dissonant stimuli. Neither condition is likely to prevail in the at-risk infant.

INTONATION. While the contouring curves for both samples are virtually identical during the newborn and 2-month period (Fig.20-3d), they diverge sharply after that. These results can best be explained by considering once again the link between contouring and affect expression and maintenance. The increasing lack of such contouring may reflect both the mother's depression in dealing with an increasingly obviously deviant child as well as the absence of the kind of cues coming from the infant and contingent upon her own behavior that allow her to remain positive and aroused. Intonation, then, seems to be a sensitive index of positive involvement at a high level of arousal.

SUMMARY

In summary then, the investigation of maternal language reveals several features important for the study of maternal behavior in general. First, the language directed to the infant differs from that directed to other adults, in that the former is less complex, more repetitious, more rhythmic, and consists of shorter vocalizations and longer pauses. On a qualitative level, it sounds unique enough to warrant consideration as a variety of "parenting behavior." Second, the emergence of features of maternal language behavior shows a developmental progression over the first 6 months of life that is well-integrated with the appearance, in the infant, of certain response capacities and preferences. Additionlly, both in degree and in pattern of emergence, these features are largely unaffected by previous maternal experience with an infant. Finally, both in the clustering of behaviors and in the level of their output, mothers of at-risk infants differ from control mothers along lines made understandable by investigation of the responsiveness of the infant and the emotional state of the mother.

Very likely, then, human infants enter onto the scene with the tendency to seek out and respond to other human beings. Other persons with whom the infant comes into contact seem especially equipped to respond to him with attention, caregiving, and a high level of positive affect. In this way, from the beginning, both the physical survival of the infant, as well as his cognitive and emotional thriving are ensured. Under optimal circumstances during the first months of life, these initial tendencies promote highly fine-tuned interactions, underscored by affective mutuality. These interchanges are not only pleasurable to parents and infants, they are of long-term consequence as well, for it is through these interactions that the infant learns the nature of communication and reciprocity that is the basis for all human relationships.

REFERENCES

Bardwick, M. Evolution and parenting. *Journal of Social Issues,* 1974, *30,*(4) 39–62.

Blount, B., & Padgug, E. Prosodic, paralinguistic and interactional features in parent-child speech: English and Spanish. *Journal of Child Language,* 1977, *4,* 67–86.

Bond, E. K. Perception of form by the human infant. *Psychological Bulletin,* 1972, *77,* 225–245.

Brazelton, T. B., Koslowski, B., & Main, M. The origins of reciprocity: The early mother-infant interaction. In M. Lewis & L. Rosenblum (Eds.). *The effect of the infant on its caregiver.* New York: Wiley, 1974.

Cann, D. Unpublished doctoral dissertation. In P. Mussen (Ed.). *Carmichael's manual of child psychology.* New York: Wiley, 1969.

Caron, A. J., Caron, R. F., Caldwell, R. C., & Weiss, S. Infant perception of the structural properties of the face. *Developmental Psychology,* 1973, *9,* 385–399.

Carpenter, G. Mother's face and the newborn, *New Scientist,* 1974, *21,* 742–744.

Cassell, Z. K., & Sander, L. W. Neonatal recognition processes and attachment: The masking experiment. Paper presented at the Society for Research in Child Development, Denver, 1975.

Chang, H., & Trehub, S. Auditory processing of relational information by young infants. *Journal of Experimental Child Psychology,* 1977, *24,* 324–331.

Charlesworth, W. R., & Kreutzer, M. A. Facial expressions of infants and children. In P. Ekman (Ed.). *Darwin and facial expression.* New York: Academic Press, 1973.

Cicchetti, D., & Sroufe, A. An organizational view of affect: Illustration from the study of Down's syndrome infants, In M. Lewis & L. Rosenblum (Eds.). *The development of affect. New York: Plenum Press, 1978.*

Condon, W. S., & Sander, L. W. Synchrony demonstrated between movements of the neonate and adult speech. *Child Development,* 1974, *45,* 456–462.

Davis, E., & Keating, J. *Mother and child.* Philadelphia: Lippincott, 1892.

Dunn, J., Wooding, C., & Hermann, J. Mother's speech to young children: Variation in context. *Developmental Medicine and Child Neurology,* 1977, *19,* 629–638.

Emde, R. N., Katz, E. L., & Thorpe, J. K. Emotional expression in infancy: II. Early deviations in Down's syndrome infants. In M. Lewis & L. Rosenblum (Eds.). *The development of affect.* New York: Plenum Press, 1978.

Fantz, R. L. Pattern vision in newborn infants. *Science,* 1963, *140,* 296–297.

Fantz, R. L. Visual perception from birth as shown by pattern selectivity. In H. E. Whipple (Ed.). *New issues in infant development. Annals of the New York Academy of Science.* 1965, *118,* 793–814.

Fantz, R. L. Visual perception and experience in early infancy: A look at the hidden side of behavior. In E. H. Hess, H. L. Rheingold & H. W. Stevenson (Eds.). *Early behavior: Comparative and developmental approaches.* New York: Wiley, 1967.

Goren, C. C., Sarty, M., & Wu, P. Y. Visual following and pattern discrimination of face-like stimuli by newborn infants. *Pediatrics,* 1975, *56,* 544–549.

Haaf, R. A., & Bell. R. Q. The facial dimension in visual discrimination by human infants. *Child Development,* 1967, *38,* 893–899.

Hershenson, M., Kessen, W., & Munsinger, H. Pattern perception in the human newborn: A closer look at some positive and negative results. In

J. C. Mott-Smith, W. Wathen-Dunn, H. Blum, & P. Lieberman (Eds.). *Symposium on models for the perception of speech and visual form.* Cambridge, Ma.: MIT Press, 1967.

Hess, E. Ethology. In A. M. Freedman & H. I. Kaplan (Eds.), *Comprehensive textbook of psychiatry.* Baltimore, Md.: Williams & Wilkins, 1967.

Hess, E. Ethology and developmental psychology. In P. Mussen (Ed.). *Carmichael's manual of child psychology.* New York: Wiley, 1969.

Hutt, S. J. Auditory discrimination at birth. In S. J. Hutt & C. Hutt (eds.). *Early human development.* Oxford, Oxford University Press, 1973.

Kearsley, R. B. The newborn's response to auditory stimulation: A demonstration of orienting and defensive behavior. *Child Development,* 1973, *44,* 582–591.

Klaus, M. H., & Kennell, J. H. *Maternal–infant bonding.* St. Louis: Mosby, 1976.

Klaus, M. H., Kennell, J. H., Plumb, N. & Zuehlke, S. Human maternal behavior at first contact with her young. *Pediatrics,* 1970, *46,* 187–192.

Kuhl, P. Speech perception in early infancy: the acquisition of speech-sound categories. In S. Hirsch, D. Eldridge, T. Hirsch, & S. Silverman (Eds.). *Hearing and Davis: Essays honoring Hollowell Davis.* St. Louis.: Washington University Press, 1976.

MacFarlane, J. A. Olfaction in the development of social preferences in the human neonate. In *Parent-Infant interaction.* Amsterdam: CIBA Foundation Symposium 33, New Series, ASP, 1975.

MacFarlane, J. A. *The psychology of childbirth,* Cambridge, Ma.: Harvard University Press, 1977.

Maurer, D., & Salapatek, P. Developmental changes in the scanning of faces by young infants. *Child Development,* 1976, *47,* 523–527.

Miranda, S. B. Visual abilities and pattern preferences of premature infants and full-term neonates. *Journal of Experimental Child Psychology,* 1970, *10,* 189–205.

Morse, P. The discrimination of speech and non-speech stimuli in early infancy. *Journal of Experimental Child Psychology,* 1972, *14,* 477–492.

Robinson, R. J. Assessment of gestational age by neurological examination. *Archives of Diseases of the Child,* 1966, *41,* 437–447.

Robson, K. The role of eye-to-eye contact in maternal-infant attachment. *Journal of Child Psychology and Psychiatry and Allied Disciplines,* 1967, *8,* 13–25.

Salk, L. The role of the heartbeat in the relationship between mother and infant. *Scientific American,* 1973, *228,* 24–29.

Sherrer, K. R. Acoustic concomitants of emotional dimensions: Judging affect from synthesized tone sequences. In S. Weitz (Ed.). *Nonverbal communication.* New York: Oxford University Press, 1974.

Snow, C. Mothers' speech to children learning language. *Child Development,* 1972, *43,* 549–565.

Snow, C. The development of conversation between mothers and babies. *Journal of Child Language,* 1977, *4,* 1–22.

Sontag, L. W., & Wallace, R. F. The movement response of the human fetus to sound stimuli. *Child Development,* 1935, *6,* 253–258.

Spelt, D. K. Conditioned responses in the human fetus in utero. *Psychological Bulletin,* 1938, *35,* 375–376.

Spelt, D. K. The conditioning of the human fetus in utero. *Journal of Experimental Psychology,* 1948, *38,* 375–376.

Spitz, R., & Wolf, M. Anaclitic depression, an inquiry into the genesis of psychiatric conditions in early childhood, II. *The Psychoanalytic Study of the Child,* 1946, *2,* 313–342.

Stern, D. N. Mother and infant at play: The dyadic interaction involving facial, vocal and gaze behaviors. In M. Lewis & L. Rosenblum (eds.). *The effect of the infants on its caregiver. New York: Wiley, 1974.*

Stern, D. N. *The first relationship: Infant and mother.* Cambridge, Ma.: Harvard University Press, 1977.

Stern, D. N., & Gibbon, J. Temporal expectancy during mother-infant play. In E. Thoman (Ed.). *Origins of the infant's social responses.* New York: Ehrlbaum Press, 1979.

Stern, D. N., Beebe, B., Jaffe, J., & Bennett, S. The infant's stimulus "world" during social interaction: A study of the structure, timing and effects of caregiver behaviors. In R. Schaffer (Ed.). *Interactions in infancy.* New York: Academic Press, 1977.

Stern, D. N., & Wasserman, G. A. Maternal language behavior to infants. Symposium presented at the society for Research in Child Development, San Francisco, 1979.

Stern, D. N., & Wasserman, G. A. The language environment of infants: The developmental role of prosodic features. In preparation.

Stern, D. N., Jaffe, J., Beebe, B., & Bennett, S. Vocalizing in unison and in alternation: Two modes of communication within the mother-infant dyad. *Annals of the New York Academy of Science,* 1975, *263,* 89–100.

Watson, J. Smiling, cooing and "the game." *Merrill-Palmer Quarterly,* 1972, *18,* 323–339

West, M. *Infant care.* United States Department of Labor, Children's Bureau. Washington, D.C.: U.S. Government Printing Office, 1914.

Wolff, P. H. Observations on the early development of smiling. In B. M. Foss (Ed.). In *Determinants of infant behavior, II.* New York: Wiley, 1963.

chapter 21

THE PREVENTION OF BIRTH TRAUMA AND INJURY THROUGH EDUCATION FOR CHILDBEARING[1]

Doris Haire

Two national perinatal studies, one carried out in the United States and the other in the United Kingdom, involving many thousands of mothers and their offspring have shown fetal hypoxia and respiratory delay at birth to be major correlates of low I.Q. and neurological impairment. Research by Ucko (1965) in England also suggests that fetal hypoxia and a delay in respiration at birth can interfere with the child's later ability to cope normally with stress, even though the child demonstrates a normal I.Q. Despite these warnings, there seems almost a world-wide effort to withhold such information from expectant mothers, as if women were too shallow to care, or unwilling to cope with the stress, discomfort, and pain of parturition in order to protect their children from the risk of such damage.

Obstetricians and anesthesiologists talk freely among

[1]This updated paper is based on a presentation made to the Fourth International Congress of the International Association for the Scientific Study of Mental Deficiency, Washington D.C, April 25, 1976.

themselves about the risks to the fetus and newborn infant of tranquilizers, analgesics, and anesthetic agents; yet, as birth draws near, American mothers are often told that there is no need to act like a martyr, that tolerating discomfort and pain during childbirth is old-fashioned. Rarely does an obstetrician discuss with an expectant mother what problems may be created for her and her child if the drugs she accepts to ease her discomfort or pain during labor and birth should cause a significant delay in her baby's ability to initiate normal respiration at birth. Effective childbirth education could fill this vacuum but all too often the information provided parents in these classes is incomplete.

If one gauges the success of a childbirth education program by the proportion of mothers who are helped to cope with the stress of childbirth without the need for drugs that depress the central nervous system, childbirth education, as it is taught in most American hospitals, is essentially a failure. Most hospital-based childbirth education classes do not deal honestly with the risks and hazards of obstetric drugs and intervention. Most nurses who teach hospital-based childbirth education classes feel compelled to provide expectant parents with only that information which the obstetricians want the parent to have, rather than teaching the parents what they need to know in order to cope with the experience and stress of labor and birth with a minimum of or no obstetric intervention and drugs.

Scott & Rose (1976) compared the infant outcome of mothers educated in the Lamaze method of childbirth and of mothers who were not so prepared. Both groups of mothers received significant amounts of obstetric medication. The investigators, using the relatively crude Apgar score, determined that there was no difference in the infant outcome of the two groups. This study is evidence that childbirth education is missing its mark when it concentrates on breathing patterns rather than on increasing the expectant mothers' tolerance of discomfort and pain by educating them to the relative risks and areas of uncertainty regarding obstetric-related drugs.

If expectant mothers were taught to refuse all obstetric practices which have not been shown by scientific, controlled evaluation to be of benefit to the obstetric patient and/or to her baby, we would see a dramatic change, and probably an improvement, in obstetric care in the United States.

The public is now being advised by various health agencies of the value of eliminating small and medium-sized obstetric services and yet, a national survey carried out by the American College of Obstetricians and Gynecologists (1970) reveals that, in general, *the larger obstetric services tend to have a greater rate of maternal and infant deaths.* The survey also showed that *the closer the affiliation between the obstetric service and a medical school the greater the rate of maternal and infant deaths.* Undoubtedly, some of these deaths result from the fact that there is a greater incidence of high-risk mothers cared for in larger teaching hospitals, but it is also possible that the greater tendency to intervene in the normal progress of labor and birth in these institutions, in order to provide experience for students, contributes to these statistics and may also result in a disproportionately high incidence of neurologically damaged children.

I do not suggest that we return to home births for all mothers. There are growing indications, however, that only by including properly organized domiciliary obstetric services for low-risk obstetric patients in regionalized obstetric programs will we learn what is the best management for low-risk mothers and their offspring. A British perinatal study (Chamberlain, 1970) showed that the lowest incidence of respiratory delay occurred among infants born at home. A study of low-risk mothers and their offspring, carried out by the California State Department of Health, revealed that the incidence of mental retardation among the home-born children (and the home-born group included those babies booked for a home birth but delivered in the hospital) was one-fifteenth that of the national average, and that the rate of cerebral palsy was one-tenth that of the national average.

Are common American hospital-based obstetric practices detrimental? Undoubtedly they contribute to the fact that one in every 35 children born in the United States today is found to be retarded, according to the National Association of Retarded Children and that in 75 percent of these cases there is no genetic or familial predisposing factor. One in every 10 to 17 children in the United States has been found to have some form of significant learning dysfunction. Such dysfunction is not limited to the poor but cuts across the entire socioeconomic and ethnic strata of American society.

Health professionals, on the whole, tend to blame our high incidence of neurologically impaired and learning disabled children only on the incidence of undernutrition, low birth weight, and prematurity—conditions more frequently found among the black population. There is a growing amount of statistical data, however, indicating that there are other factors involved. An extensive survey by Gruenwald (1976) indicated that 40 to 60 percent of all perinatal deaths occurred among newborn infants who weighed over 5½ pounds and who were close to or at full-term. A more recent report (Drorbaugh et al., 1975) on the Boston component of the federally funded Collaborative Perinatal Study, indicates that 80 percent of the 7-year-old children found to have abnormal or suspect central nervous system functions were of normal weight at birth.

Unfortunately, we cannot look to the 150 million dollar Collaborative Perinatal Study to guide us to a safe form of analgesia or anesthesia, nor to the best way to manage labor and birth, for the study did not include a sufficient control group of healthy, unmedicated mothers and their offspring who could have served as a baseline against which to measure deviations from normal newborn infant behavior and response. Virtually all of the healthy women in the Collaborative Perinatal Study received drugs during labor and/or birth. The results of the study were further skewed by the fact that obstetric intervention, such as forceps extraction, etc., were more frequently carried out on the healthy parturients in the study—the group more likely to produce healthy children—while obstetric intervention tended to be avoided among the high-risk mothers in order to spare those fetuses, already in jeopardy, from further trauma.

The fact that black women, at least during the time the study was carried out, were frequently denied pain-relieving drugs and time-consuming intervention was undoubtedly a blessing in disguise. A follow-up review by Niswander and Gordon (1972) reports that *among the over 50,000 children evaluated at 1 year of age there was an unexpected, slightly greater incidence of significant brain damage among the white children at one year of age than among the black children of the same age.* Table 21–1 summarizes these findings.

I must add, however, that by the time the black children in the study reached the age of 4 social deprivation and undernutrition had taken its toll, and the statistics were reversed, but the better outcome of the black children at 1 year of age is there for all to see and ponder.

There is no question that medically indicated obstetric drugs have saved thousands of lives, but that does not excuse the fact that millions of unborn children have been exposed during their intrauterine existence to unnecessary drugs— drugs that have been released or approved by the United States Food and Drug Administration as safe for use by childbearing women. Yet, according to the Committee on Drugs of the American Academy of Pediatrics (1973), *there is no drug, whether prescription drug or over-the-counter remedy, which has been proven safe for the unborn child.* Few expectant parents are advised by their obstetrician or pediatrician of the opinion of this learned group. This indicates that childbirth education, which fails to discuss the areas of uncertainty concerning obstetric drugs, fails to protect the interest of the unseen obstetric patient—the unborn child.

While there are indications that attitudes towards drugs are changing, nausea remedies, diuretics, laxatives, appetite suppressants, etc., are still being prescribed for pregnant

Table 21–1 Collaborative Perinatal Study
National Institute of Neurologic Diseases and Blindness

Neurologic outcome by race	White			Black		
Outcomes	No. of cases	Number	Rate per 1000	No. of cases	Number	Rate per 1000
Births	19,048			20,167		
Perinatal deaths		688	35.07		845	41.90
Stillbirths		415	21.79		457	22.66
Fresh stillbirths		200	10.50		246	12.20
Live births	18,633			19,710		
Neonatal deaths		253	13.58		388	19.69
Live births with known birth weight	18,481*			19,504†		
Birth weight under 2501 gm		1319	71.37		2617	134.18
One year exams	14,662			17,123		
Neurologically abnormal at 1 yr.		253	17.26		274	16.00

*Mean Birth Weight: 3273 grams
†Mean Birth Weight: 3039 grams

women. Antacids, antispasmodics, uterine stimulants, seda-
tives, tranquilizers, muscle relaxants, amnesiacs, narcotics,
analgesics, regional anesthesia, and inhalation anesthesia have
become so routine in American obstetric care that most health
professionals and parents have tended to grow complacent
about the common use of these drugs during labor and birth.
Yet we do not know whether any of these drugs administered
singly or in combinations permanently affect the mental and
neurologic development of the child exposed to these drugs in
utero. Experts in pharmacology remind us that the most dangerous drugs and chemicals in our environment are those which
cannot be sensed by humans. Diethylstilbestrol (DES) for example, caused no apparent alteration in fetal heart rate or alteration in maternal blood pressure as it did its damage.

As new techniques become available for testing the effects
of obstetric drugs and procedures on the fetus and newborn
infant, it becomes increasingly apparent that parents, as well as
professionals, must reevaluate the wisdom of common American obstetric practices. Fifty mg of meperidine given to the
mother during labor—once considered an innocuous dose—has
now been shown to cause respiratory depression in one out of
every four newborn infants.

With all of our technology, no one knows the degree of
maternal hypotension or oxygen depletion that an unborn or
newborn infant can tolerate before he or she sustains permanent
brain damage, dysfunction, or death. Nor do we know the
long-term effects of electively inducing or chemically stimulat-
ing labor contractions, artificially rupturing the amniotic membranes, confining the mother to bed during labor, applying
fundal pressure, or extracting a baby by forceps. Considering
how little we know, is it wise to administer a pudendal block
to a woman about to deliver? This block can alter the fetal
heartrate and inhibit the mother's ability to give birth spontaneously.

Abouleish (1975) explains that injecting the anesthetic
agent for pudendal block into the vagina is not painful because

the area is numbed by the pressure from the fetal head. In light of this fact, why give the injections *before* the baby is born? If necessary for episiotomy repair, the injections can be given *after* the baby is born while the perineal area is still numb and the baby cannot be adversely affected by the anesthetic agent.

Anesthesiologists are now recommending epidural anesthesia as a means of avoiding the adverse effects of maternal stress during labor and birth. Yet they have not investigated whether tender care and strong emotional support and encouragement might be a more effective and a safer means of maintaining the delicate balance of maternal-fetal physiology.

There is currently a concerted effort by many health professionals to push epidural blocks as the "Cadillac of anesthetics." Tronick et al. (1976) found that epidural anesthesia has no adverse effects on "highly selected" babies. In that study, however, any infant who had a problem in the delivery room, such as a delay in respiration, marked acrocyanosis, hypothermia, (all conditions that can be precipitated or intensified by the use of drugs used in epidural block) was omitted. Furthermore, any deviations from the accepted standard of normal newborn behavior or condition in the nursery were further grounds for exclusion. It is not surprising that the authors obtained such a favorable outcome from such a "stacked deck" of prescreened infants. It is somewhat analogous to saying,

> Having limited our study to a select group of healthy soldiers who survived the war without trauma or injury, we are pleased to report that none of the select group showed any adverse effects from having been in combat.

Those who would justify the routine use of drugs during labor and birth on the grounds that the electronic monitor will identify deviations in normal fetal physiology should be reminded of or alerted to the fact that *no one knows the long-term or delayed effects of ultrasound, used in electronic fetal monitors,*

on the later physical, neurologic, and mental development of the
child in utero or on the delicate ovum of the female fetus.

A review of the research (Banta & Thacker, 1979) on
electronic fetal monitoring (EFM) has shown that it does *not*
contribute to improved infant outcome among low-risk women
and that there *are definite risks* to this costly and widely used
technology. The authors of the report, Dr. David Banta, Health
Programs Manager, Office of Technology Assessment, Congress of the United States and Dr. Stephen Thacker, Chief,
Consolidated Surveillance and Communication Activity, Bureau of Epidemiology, Center for Disease Control, suggest the
need for more careful evaluation and control of medical tech-
nologies. The U.S. Food and Drug Administration (FDA) has
heeded their cautions by recommending that pregnant women
not be exposed to EFM unless the medical information to be
gained is essential and clearly worth the known risks, including
the risk stemming from the uncertainty as to the delayed long-
term effects of ultrasound. The FDA has recommended that
pregnant women should not be used as models to demonstrate
ultrasonic devices. Those who still contend that ultrasound
used for fetal monitoring is harmless also should be reminded
that many men and women now have iatrogenic cancer as a
result of x-ray therapy for acne, enlarged tonsils, etc. which at
the time x-ray therapy was used, was considered harmless.

Dr. Caldeyro-Barcia (1979), President of the International
Federation of Obstetricians and Gynecologists, recently cautioned that confining the mother to bed during labor, in order
to maintain the position of the external fetal monitor, tended
to alter the normal fetal environment.

In most countries other than the United States, women are
encouraged to walk during labor in order to lessen the mother's
discomfort and to assure the normal progress of labor. Controlled research by Flynn et al. (1978) has demonstrated that
those women who are encouraged to walk about during labor
have significantly shorter labors (by more than 2 hours), significantly less need for drugs to relieve their discomfort or pain,

and, in turn, fewer but more effective contractions. The infants of mothers who were confined to bed during labor were more than five times more likely to be delivered by forceps. They also experienced significantly more nonnormal fetal heart rate patterns during labor and had poorer Apgar scores at 1 minute and 5 minutes after birth than did the infants of those mothers who were encouraged to walk during labor.

Caldeyro-Barcia and his colleagues have also warned against and demonstrated several adverse effects resulting from amniotomy (artificial rupture of the amniotic sac) during labor. Most of these adverse effects result from the fact that amniotomy disturbs the normal balance of pressure received by the uterine contents (the fetus, placenta, and umbilical cord), during contractions and the bearing down period. The loss of this hydraulic "cushion" increases the likelihood of uneven compression and deformation of the fetal head, which, in turn, jeopardizes the fetal brain because of the increased probability of a rupture in the membranes which surround and support the fetal brain, with resultant intracranial hemorrhage. There is also an increased likelihood that the umbilical cord will become compressed to the point of occlusion by the powerful contracting uterine muscles altering the infant's supply of oxygen and otherwise changing the chemistry of the fetal blood.

It has become increasingly evident that the so-called judicious use of obstetric drugs and procedures can only be determined after the child is born, when it may be too late to correct an error in judgment. The fallacy of judging the safety of a drug or procedure only by its short-term effects has been made tragically evident by the fact that DES, given to millions of pregnant American women in order to forestall premature labor, has now been linked statistically to a significantly increased incidence of cancer and abnormalities of the reproductive system in female offspring 10 to 20 years after exposure to the drug in utero (AAP, 1973). The increased incidence of abnormalities of the reproductive tract in the male offspring of mothers given DES during their pregnancies is now becoming evident. It has taken us 20 years to discover the latent effects of hormonal therapy for expectant mothers on their offspring. There are now indications that hormones administered to pregnant women may later affect the sexual behavior of their adult offspring. How can we possibly begin to evaluate the effect of obstetric drugs on the exposed offspring's later mental and neurologic development if the mother's prenatal and intranatal records are permitted to be destroyed before the child reaches the age of adulthood? Unfortunately, such destruction of records is now permitted in many states in the United States.

It is not difficult to understand how the present state of complacency regarding obstetric-related drugs came about. Many physicians practicing today received their training at a time when the placenta was still viewed as a protective barrier, preventing the drugs administered to the mother from entering the fetal circulation in any significant quantity. Although we now know that the placenta is not a barrier but, in the words of the late Virginia Apgar, a "bloody sieve," old ideas die hard.

An example of misinformation which lingers on beyond its time is evident in "Obstetric Anesthesia and Analgesia" a booklet available from the American College of Obstetricians and Gynecologists (1969). One sentence reads: "I personally am in favor of using a regional anesthetic whenever possible, principally because it does not ordinarily enter the blood stream and cannot reach the baby's system." One would hardly expect to find this erroneous information being perpetuated. In addition, the booklet also refers to an infant who has been affected by his mother's obstetric drugs as "sleepy," rather than drugged. The book ends with the statement, "With the many analgesic and anesthetic agents available, she (the mother) can expect a safe and relatively comfortable delivery."

Such assurances from an agency such as the ACOG leave the mother with a false sense of well-being. It is virtually impossible to predict how an individual mother and her unborn baby will be affected by a given obstetric drug since many physiochemical factors influence how a drug affects the mother and her unborn baby.

Another example of misinformation is the assumption of some physicians that drugs which will depress the central nervous system of women in labor will improve the fetal environment and the infant's status following birth. Such a recommendation is based on an unproven hypothesis and is frequently an extrapolation based on research by Myers & Myers (1979) which demonstrated that, when a wild monkey experiencing contractions is purposely frightened and inflicted with pain, the adrenal medulla produces an excess of hormones called catechoiamines. The sympathetic nerve reaction and the catecholamines cause the blood vessels of the monkey's uterus to constrict, causing hypoxia (oxygen deprivation) in the fetus. The authors are careful to point out that this cause and effect relationship has not been shown to be true in humans. (Nor has the same phenomenon been shown to occur in tame monkeys accustomed to human contact.) The careful reader will discern from the Myers' review the very important fact that the discomfort and pain of normal labor have not been shown to cause an increase in maternal catecholamines, nor a sympathetic nerve reaction sufficient to cause fetal or newborn hypoxia.

There is no question that obstetric drugs have saved thousands of lives and are essential to the armamentarium of the obstetrician, but the fact remains that *any* drug that artificially changes the fetal environment or the mother's or fetus's blood chemistry can jeopardize the fetus and the integrity of the fetal brain. For example, oxytocin, administered to a mother to induce labor and/or to accelerate labor, can impede the oxygenation of the fetus by increasing the length and intensity of the contractions beyond the physiologically normal range, and by artificially shortening the intervals *between* contractions. During a contraction, when the mother's flow of oxygenated blood to the placenta is constricted or "pinched off" by the contracting uterine wall, the baby's brain is supplied with oxygen from the oxygenated blood stored up in the placenta *between* contractions. Interfering with this vital process can result in brain damage or death.

Any drug that slows the mother's respiration or lowers her blood pressure or increases the need to rupture the amniotic membranes can adversely affect the fetus and newborn infant. The same is true of any procedure that increases the need for fundal pressure, forceps extraction, cesarean section, or resuscitation of the newborn infant. Surely it is irresponsible to subject the fetus to any unnecessary procedure or drug which can possibly alter the functioning of so complex and vital an organ as the human brain. Yet, childbirth education classes held in hospitals, tend to promote the idea that, in the hands of a qualified anesthesiologist, analgesics and anesthetic agents are perfectly safe for the fetus. No one yet knows the degree of drug toxicity, oxygen depletion, fundal pressure, head compression or traction by forceps that an unborn infant can tolerate before he sustains permanent brain damage.

Brackbill (1974, 1976) cautioned that the human baby is particularly susceptible to the damaging effects of obstetric drugs because at the time of birth the newborn infant's brain is structurally and functionally incomplete. Because the brain of the fetus and newborn infant is undergoing very rapid change and growth these intricate developing neurological systems are more susceptible to permanent damage. Brackbill has cautioned that environmental influences can change the direction in which these systems develop, the rate at which they develop, and even the extent to which they develop at all. After the baby is born and must depend on his own bodily functions to detoxify drugs remaining in his system after birth, the rapidly developing nervous system is even more vulnerable to environmental insults that will reroute or alter the neurological development of the child. Further, Brackbill warns that many drugs appear to be, in a sense, trapped in the brain and are detoxified only after a relatively long period of time. For example, Valium administered to mothers during labor can still be found in the tissues of their newborn infants 10 days after birth.

Dr. Peter Auld, Professor of Pediatrics and Director of Nurseries for New York Hospital-Cornell Medical Center, has warned that we cannot consider the positive evaluation of a newborn infant, via the Apgar Score, immediately following birth, as an assurance of infant well-being. Auld cautions that an infant on the verge of going into shock can exhibit an Apgar Score of 8 or 9. Aleksandrowicz and Aleksandrowicz (1974) point out that adverse responses to obstetric drugs, such as secondary depression or impaired sucking reflex, may not become evident for several hours following birth.

Blue hands and feet are seen so frequently in American hospital-born infants after the first hour of life that parents are now told in most hospital-based childbirth education classes that such a condition is normal. In commenting on the frequency of this condition among American newborn infants, Dr. Albert Huch, obstetrician-physiologist from the University of Marburg, Germany, recently said, "Yes, you Americans consider blue hands and feet after the first few minutes of life to be normal, but we do not consider a baby in that condition to be in optimal condition." Therein lies the difference. While American health professionals tend to be satisfied with the "average" or "normal" baby, health professionals in those countries that have a better infant outcome tend to put their efforts into seeing that every baby is in optimal condition at birth.

We have much to learn from such countries as the Netherlands where, based on all available evidence, respiratory delay is rare even in high-risk obstetric units, and the rates of neurologic impairment and mental deficiency are significantly less than in the United States. Obviously, the causes of mental deficiency are multifactorial, but there is no doubt, in my mind, that obstetric drugs that interfere with the normal progress of labor and birth and the immediate respiration of the newborn contribute to the skyrocketing incidence of mental retardation and learning disability in the United States, and that changing our present system of obstetric care would reduce this incidence.

Despite the potential danger that maternal hypotension poses to the fetal brain, a drop in maternal blood pressure resulting from obstetric drugs has become so common among American obstetric patients that in many instances hypotension is not noted on the mother's labor and delivery record, unless the drop is significant. But what is a "significant" drop in maternal blood pressure in regard to the fetal brain? How much of a drop in maternal blood pressure can occur before the transfer of oxygen from the mother to the fetus is so reduced that the fetal brain is permanently damaged? Unfortunately, no one knows. A vasopressor drug can be administered to the mother to increase her blood pressure but there is no assurance that the blood flow to the uterus will return to normal quickly enough to avoid damage to the fetal brain.

Hoffman (1971) found that when the health histories of children who were failing in school were compared with those of children who were performing satisfactorily there were significant differences in the birth histories of the two groups of children. Prematurity did appear to play a role in learning impairment, being five times more common among the learning-impaired children than among the children doing satisfactory work in school. Prematurity, however, was a comparatively minor factor, when compared to the incidence of difficult delivery, cyanosis (oxygen deprivation), and prolonged labor. Prolonged labor and cyanosis in the newborn occurred 20 times more often among the births of those children who were failing in school. Difficult delivery, also precipitated or aggravated by the administration of common obstetric drugs, occurred 16 times more often among the births of those children who were failing in school. Figure 21–1 summarizes Hoffman's results. It is interesting to note that Hoffman found that induced labor put the baby in the same category of risk as those babies who were products of prematurity, breech delivery, and

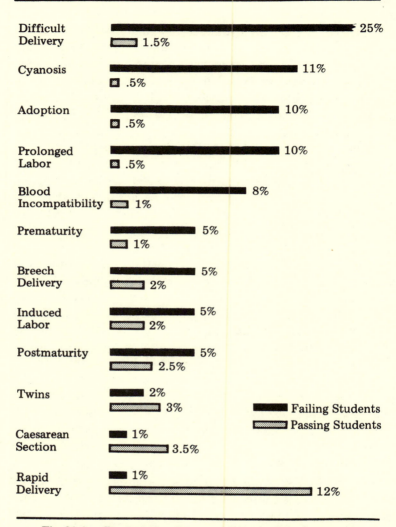

Fig. 21-1. Comparisons of the perinatal histories of failing and passing students. From Hoffman, M. Early indication of learning disabilities. *Academic Therapy,* 1971, *1,* 2–26.

postmaturity, conditions one would not inflict on a baby if at all possible to avoid. Other studies have supported her results. These findings should make it apparent that, whenever possible, we must employ means other than obstetric drugs of minimizing the mother's discomfort or pain.

Much of the complacency regarding drugs has undoubtedly resulted from the fact that all of them have been released or approved for use by the FDA, with no restrictions regarding their use by childbearing women. Yet, Dr. Richard Crout, Director of the Bureau of Drugs of the U. S. Food and Drug Administration, has confirmed in writing that (1) *the FDA does not guarantee the safety of any drug it releases or approves as safe and effective;* and that (2) the criteria used by the FDA for determining the safety of drugs administered to women during labor and birth *has not and does not include a requirement that the long-term safety be shown for the mental and neurological development of the child exposed to the drug in utero.*

In most cases, the FDA does not require a manufacturer to test the interaction of his drug in conjunction with other drugs likely to be used for the same condition before approving the drug as safe. The FDA, in fact, has no specific definition for "safe."

Prior to the 1962 amendments to the Food, Drug and Cosmetic Act (the period of time in which most of the drugs presently being used in obstetrics came on the market,) the FDA had no power to actually approve a drug as safe for use or marketing. The FDA had only the authority to announce a new drug application, wait 30 to 60 days, and if there were no serious objections to the drug's use, the application was approved. Even today a drug may be marketed without a new drug application being filed with the FDA if the drug is essentially the same as an "old" drug that has been on the market for many years, even though that old drug has never been scientifically investigated and shown to be safe. There are many drugs presently being given to obstetric patients that have never been officially reviewed, released, or approved for use by the FDA. Once a drug is on the market it is rarely taken off. Certainly, it is unlikely that subtle neurological damage would be traced to obstetric-related drugs, and even less likely that the damage would be reported to the FDA under our present system. One of the reasons for this is that there is no law requiring a physician to report an adverse drug reaction to the FDA. Such reporting is strictly voluntary. Even if a law is passed to require the reporting of an adverse reaction to a *new* drug, this will not affect our knowledge of the hundreds of obstetric drugs already on the market.

By not requiring the manufacturer of a drug or medical device to include a clear warning that the product has not been proven safe for the unborn child, the FDA has allowed the manufacturer to delude the consumer into assuming that the product has been proven safe since, after all, it has been released or approved as "safe" by the FDA. Nor does the FDA require the manufacturer to warn the user of the more obtuse but pertinent facts about a given medication and its indirect effect on the fetus whenever administered to the pregnant or parturient woman. For example, drug-induced uterine inertia may precipitate the need for the chemical stimulation of labor, the artificial rupture of membranes to speed labor, the application of fundal pressure and forceps extractions to speed up delivery —all procedures that can create additional trauma to the brain of the unborn child. Yet, when one reads the package insert sheet there is no mention that the use of a given drug will increase the need for these procedures, even when the warning is applicable.

It is unfortunate that, in most states, hospitals are not required to attach a complete copy of the mother's prenatal, intranatal, and postnatal records to the infant's record in order that this important information be available for future reference or study. Physicians, psychologists, and other therapists who request such records are frequently offered only a summary or abstract of the mother's records. Unfortunately, a summary or abstract of the mother's records frequently omits information that might be of value to the child's therapist in later years. Microfilmed records are all too often illegible and, according to FBI document experts, will not always reveal alterations in the original records.

In many states, such as Illinois, Michigan, and Georgia, there is no requirement that hospitals preserve the mother's record beyond her hospital stay. In addition, most states permit the immediate destruction of nurses' notes, which could provide valuable information to investigators as to the hour-to-hour state of the mother and fetus during labor and birth. The tragedy of the destruction of the mother's prenatal, intranatal, and postnatal records is that the information in these destroyed records could help scientists to identify those drugs that can affect the neurological and mental development of the children exposed to the drugs in utero.

CONCLUSION

A recent report to the United States Congress by the Comptroller General's Office (September 24, 1979) stated that, based on investigation, more coordinated federal and private efforts are needed to evaluate the benefits and risks of obstetric practices. It further stated that there is still insufficient evaluation of the safety of obstetric procedures. The physician has a legal obligation to obtain the mother's informed consent prior to treatment. Therefore, the physician must advise the expectant mother not only of the benefits of the various obstetric drugs and procedures but also of the risk—including the risk of uncertainty regarding the delayed, long term effects of the drugs and procedures on the subsequent development of the offspring. Such knowledge is crucial to prospective parents who wish to participate actively and responsibly in these decisions involving the mother's obstetric care and the care of their newborn infant. This information might well be provided in child-birth education classes as well as in health science classes. If healthy child development is our goal, research on the effects of obstetric practices and complete dissemination of facts and data is essential.

REFERENCES

Abouleish, E. *Childbirth is a joy not a suffering.* Philadelphia: Dorrance, 1975.

Aleksandrowicz, M. K. & Aleksandrowicz, D. The effect of pain relieving drugs administered during labor and delivery on the behavior of the newborn. *Merrill-Palmer Quarterly,* 1974, *20,* 121–141.

American Academy of Pediatrics Committee on Drugs. Stilbestrol and adenocarcinoma of the vagina. *Pediatrics,* 1973, *51,* 297–99.

American College of Obstetrics and Gynecology. Obstetric anesthesia and analgesia during childbirth. *AGOC Technical Bulletin,* 1969, *11.*

American College of Obstetrics and Gynecology Committee on Maternal Health. *National study of maternity care survey of obstetric practice and associated service in hospitals in the United States.* Chicago: AGOC, 1970.

Banta, H. D. & Thacker, S. The premature delivery of medical technology. *Ob/Gyn Survey,* 1979, special supplement, *34* (8), 627–642.

Brackbill, Y. Obstetric premedication and infant outcome. *American Journal of Obstetrics and Gynecology,* 1976, *118,* 377–388.

Brackbill, Y. Oral presentation. American Foundation for Maternal and Child Health. New York, March, 1974.

Caldeyro-Barcia, R. The influence of maternal position during the second stage of labor. Presentation, Ninth International Congress, International Federation of Obstetrics and Gynecology, Tokyo, 1979.

Chamberlain, R. *British births, 1970, vol. 1: The first week of life.* London: Medical Books, 1976.

Comptroller General of the United States, Report to Congress. Evaluation of benefits and risks of obstetric practices—more coordinated federal and private efforts needed. United States publication number HRD 7985. General Accounting Office, Sept. 24, 1979.

Drorbaugh, J., Moore, D., & Warren, J. Association between gestational and environmental events and central nervous system function in seven year old children. *Pediatrics,* 1975, *56,* 529–537.

FDA, *Diagnostic ultrasound equipment*. Federal Register, February, 1979, 44, (31), 9542–9544.

FDA, *Considerations general considerations for the clinical evaluation of drugs in infants and children*, HEW/FDA, 77, 3041.

Flynn, A., Kelly, J., Hollins, G. & Lynch, P. Ambulation during labor. *British Medical Journal*, 1978, *6, 37,* 591–593.

Gruenwald, P. Perinatal death of full-sized and full-term babies. *American Journal of Obstetrics and Gynecology*, 1976, *107,* 1022–1030.

Hoffman, M. Early indications of learning problems. *Academic Therapy*, 1971, *7,* 23–35.

Myers, R. & Myers, S. Use of sedative, analgesic, and anesthesic drugs during labor and delivery: Bane or boom. *American Journal of Obstetrics and Gynecology*, 1979, *133,* 83–104.

Niswander, K. & Gordon, M. Women and their pregnancies: *The collaborative perinatal study of the national institute of neurological diseases and stroke.* Philadelphia: Saunders, 1972.

Scott, J. & Rose, N. Effect of psychoprophylaxis (Lamaze preparation) on labor and delivery. *New England Journal of Medicine*, 1976, *294,* 1205–1207.

Tronick, E., Wise, S., Heidelise, A., Adamson, L., Scanlon, J., Brazelton, B. Regional obstetric anesthesia and newborn behavior: Effect over the first ten days of life. *Pediatrics*, 1976, *58,* 95–100.

Ucko, L. A comparative study of asphyxiated and non-asphyxiated boys from birth to five years. *Developmental Medical Child Neurology*, 1965, *7,* 643–657.

INDEX